D0264003

PRAISE FOR

Maximise Your Health with the Blood Type Diet

r. D'Adamo's revolutionary program, his development
Blood-Type Diet, has quite simply changed my life. It's
me a baseline from which to go forward—and a way
f t   iting that makes sense. His work has put me back on
ding edge of my life, both mentally and physically. I'd
end it to anyone searching to reclaim their well-being."

— **Andrew McCarthy**, actor/director

"When a colleague handed me a packet of information
about the D'Adamo Institute for the Advancement of Natural
Therapies, I weighed nearly 200 pounds after a year on high-dose
steroids, drugs that were treating my autoimmune disease but
taking a toll on my body. Even when my doctors found another
less toxic drug, they cautioned me to have modest expectations of
weig it loss, reminding me that I was postmenopausal. By following
Dr.   's instructions, I lost 70 pounds, 10 more than I had gained;
s vly reduced my medication by 60 percent; and many days
feel fantastic. There is much wisdom in his advice."

— **Denise M. Nagel, M.D.**

30131 05033508 9

LONDON BOROUGH OF BARNET

MAXIMISE YOUR HEALTH
with the Blood Type Diet

Also by Dr. James L. D'Adamo

THE D'ADAMO DIET

ONE MAN'S FOOD . . . is someone else's poison
(with Allan Richards)

Hay House Titles of Related Interest

YOU CAN HEAL YOUR LIFE, the movie,
starring Louise L. Hay & Friends
(available as a 1-DVD program and an expanded 2-DVD set)
Watch the trailer at: **www.LouiseHayMovie.com**

THE SHIFT, the movie,
starring Dr. Wayne W. Dyer
(available as a 1-DVD program and an expanded 2-DVD set)
Watch the trailer at: **www.DyerMovie.com**

RAW BASICS: Incorporating Raw Living Foods into Your Diet Using Easy and Delicious Recipes, by Jenny Ross

HEALTH BLISS: 50 Revitalizing NatureFoods & Lifestyle Choices to Promote Vibrant Health, by Susan Smith Jones, Ph.D.

HEAL YOUR BODY: The Mental Causes for Physical Illness and the Metaphysical Way to Overcome Them, by Louise L. Hay

UNLOCK THE SECRET MESSAGES OF YOUR BODY! A 28-Day Jump-Start Program for Radiant Health and Glorious Vitality, by Denise Linn

THE VITAMIN D REVOLUTION: How the Power of This Amazing Vitamin Can Change Your Life, by Soram Khalsa, M.D.

Please visit:

Hay House UK: **www.hayhouse.co.uk**
Hay House USA: **www.hayhouse.com**®
Hay House Australia: **www.hayhouse.com.au**
Hay House South Africa: **www.hayhouse.co.za**
Hay House India: **www.hayhouse.co.in**

MAXIMISE YOUR HEALTH

with the Blood Type Diet

A REVOLUTIONARY PLAN TO ACHIEVE OPTIMUM WELLNESS

Dr James L. D'Adamo
With Allan Richards

HAY HOUSE

Australia • Canada • Hong Kong • India
South Africa • United Kingdom • United States

First published and distributed in the United Kingdom by:
Hay House UK Ltd, 292B Kensal Rd, London W10 5BE. Tel.: (44) 20 8962 1230;
Fax: (44) 20 8962 1239. www.hayhouse.co.uk

Published and distributed in the United States of America by:
Hay House, Inc., PO Box 5100, Carlsbad, CA 92018-5100. Tel.: (1) 760 431 7695
or (800) 654 5126; Fax: (1) 760 431 6948 or (800) 650 5115. www.hayhouse.com

Published and distributed in Australia by:
Hay House Australia Ltd, 18/36 Ralph St, Alexandria NSW 2015. Tel.: (61) 2 9669
4299; Fax: (61) 2 9669 4144. www.hayhouse.com.au

Published and distributed in the Republic of South Africa by:
Hay House SA (Pty), Ltd, PO Box 990, Witkoppen 2068. Tel./Fax: (27) 11 467
8904. www.hayhouse.co.za

Published and distributed in India by:
Hay House Publishers India, Muskaan Complex, Plot No.3, B-2, Vasant Kunj, New
Delhi – 110 070. Tel.: (91) 11 4176 1620; Fax: (91) 11 4176 1630.
www.hayhouse.co.in

Distributed in Canada by:
Raincoast, 9050 Shaughnessy St, Vancouver, BC V6P 6E5. Tel.: (1) 604 323 7100;
Fax: (1) 604 323 2600

Copyright © 2010 by James L. D'Adamo

The moral rights of the authors have been asserted.

Editorial supervision: Jill Kramer • *Project editor:* Lisa Mitchell
Design: Tricia Breidenthal

All of the stories and case studies in this book are true; however, all names have
been changed for confidentiality purposes.

All rights reserved. No part of this book may be reproduced by any mechanical,
photographic or electronic process, or in the form of a phonographic recording;
nor may it be stored in a retrieval system, transmitted or otherwise be copied for
public or private use, other than for 'fair use' as brief quotations embodied in
articles and reviews, without prior written permission of the publisher.

The authors of this book do not dispense medical advice or prescribe the use of
any technique as a form of treatment for physical or medical problems without
the advice of a physician, either directly or indirectly. The intent of the authors
is only to offer information of a general nature to help you in your quest for
emotional and spiritual wellbeing. In the event you use any of the information
in this book for yourself, which is your constitutional right, the authors and the
publisher assume no responsibility for your actions.

A catalogue record for this book is available from the British Library.

ISBN 978-1-84850-589-6

Printed and bound in Great Britain by TJ International, Padstow, Cornwall.

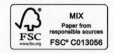

*This book is dedicated to my loving wife,
Christiana, who has always been there for me,
allowing me the time to continue in my research.
I never could have written this without her.*

CONTENTS

FOREWORD

by Louise L. Hay

Life has so many interesting twists and turns.

If only we were taught as children that prevention is the best way to maintain vibrant health. Instead, we're inundated with glossy, cheerful ads for processed, sugary junk foods . . . foods that are purposely addictive and detrimental to our health.

Then in time, our bodies react to this lack of good, natural nutrition; and we discover that we've contracted assorted diseases. It's so much easier to keep a healthy body healthy than to have to repair a body that has gone downhill.

That was my story until I was diagnosed with cancer more than 30 years ago.

You can imagine my surprise and delight when I received a letter from Dr. D'Adamo in the spring of 2009. I was smiling with joy as I opened it. Positive memories flooded back to me as I remembered the man who had taught me so much about health.

As I read the beginning of the letter: "As a former patient of mine, publisher, and advocate of alternative health care, I would very much appreciate it if you were to publish this book. . . ." I leaped to my feet, thinking, *Yes, of course, I would—in a New York minute!* After all this man had done for me, I felt grateful to be able to do something special for *him.*

As I mentioned, I was diagnosed with cancer three decades ago. With my background of being raped at the age of five and being a battered child who was sexually abused for many years, it was no wonder I manifested cancer in the vaginal area.

Yes, it frightened me; however, I had been studying and teaching self-healing for several years, so here was Life giving me the opportunity to prove to myself that what I'd been teaching really worked. After all, I'd written the book on the mental patterns for dis-eases in the body (*Heal Your Body*), and I knew that cancer was a dis-ease stemming from deep resentment that has been held for a long time until it literally eats away at the body.

I truly believed that the word *incurable,* which is so frightening to so many people, meant to me that this particular condition could not be cured by any outer means and that it was necessary to go *within* to find the cure.

I immediately took responsibility for my own healing and embarked on a journey of discovery. I read and investigated everything I could find on alternative, holistic ways to assist my healing process. I learned that I needed to release resentment; practice forgiveness; and engage in processes such as foot reflexology, colon therapy, and other methodologies. I was also told that it was vital to find a good nutritionist.

Life somehow brought me to Dr. James D'Adamo. The most important part of my healing journey had arrived.

I learned several things from this experience. First: Trust Life. No matter how dire the circumstances seem to be, there is always a solution, a way out. The foods we choose to eat and the thoughts we choose to think have *everything* to do with our health. Junk foods and negative thoughts simply destroy our health. The body knows how to heal itself; we just need to supply it with the nutrition it needs.

Today I am in my 80s, am blessed with energy, and still maintain the beneficial practices that Dr. James D'Adamo recommended to me so many years ago. I give enormous thanks to him for all he has taught me about how to bring my body back to vibrant health. It worked for me, and it can work for you.

There are times in life when someone does you an enormous favor and you wonder how you could ever pay it back. Well, now I know.

May you benefit from this wise man's knowledge!

INTRODUCTION

Nearly 30 years ago, Dr. James D'Adamo and I collaborated on *One Man's Food . . . is someone else's poison,* the original book about Dr. D'Adamo's groundbreaking work on the correlation between blood types and diet. Since our book first appeared in 1980, Dr. D'Adamo's son, Dr. Peter D'Adamo, wrote *Eat Right 4 Your Type,* in which he acknowledges *One Man's Food* and his father's concept of individualized treatment based on blood types as the source of his work.

As I wrote in the Introduction to *One Man's Food,* my then wife Ingrid Boulting introduced me to Dr. James D'Adamo. Ingrid and I were newly married, and her wedding present to me was a one-hour trip on the subway from our apartment in Manhattan to Dr. D'Adamo's office in Bay Ridge, Brooklyn. I put up a fuss about seeing him—I was a '60s guy who had heard the slogan "You are what you eat" often enough to pay attention to it. I favored a Mediterranean-style diet of fish, vegetables, and pastas and didn't get sick much, so why did I need to see him? What was so special about him?

What distinguished Dr. D'Adamo, Ingrid argued, was the fact that he created individualized diets and physical regimens—lifestyles based on a person's blood type: O, A, B, or AB—and she insisted I was going to see him. Although highly skeptical, I relented and journeyed to his office. There I sat for over an hour in a crowded waiting room. Once summoned to meet Dr. D'Adamo, I was diagnosed by a method he called iridology—he claimed that the iris of the eye is like a map of the entire body and registers weaknesses in the organs and can detect developing diseases. After reading my eyes and noting which organs were compromised or damaged—"your kidneys and liver are fatigued," he blithely reported—he pricked my finger, smeared a drop of my blood on a slide, and tested my blood type. I was a B. That's all he needed, he said. He then spent the next 45 minutes creating a specific menu, listing every fruit, vegetable, grain, dairy product, and animal protein I could eat, and those I definitely needed to avoid.

That encounter led to a change in my lifestyle, making me even more health conscious, and, ultimately, to the collaboration with Dr. D'Adamo. After *One Man's Food* was published, Dr. D'Adamo moved to Toronto, where he opened a naturopathic institute and practiced for 20 years; and then to Portsmouth, New Hampshire, a charming New England city where he established the D'Adamo Institute for the Advancement of Natural Therapies. I eventually moved to the Miami area.

Dr. D'Adamo Calls

Several months ago while I was walking toward my office at Florida International University in North Miami where I teach journalism, Ingrid called. The conversation went as follows:

"Hi Allan, it's Ingrid. How are you?"

"Fine, how are you? I can't speak, I'm rushing—"

(Ignoring the urgency) "Dr. D'Adamo called . . . he's looking for you."

(Stopped in my tracks) "D'Adamo? What does he want?!"

"He wants you to write his next book. He couldn't find you, so he looked me up on the Internet."

"Write his next book? I haven't heard from him in 30 years and I should write his next book?! I'm late for a meeting—"

"Here's his number; he wants you to call him. . . ."

But I didn't call. A few weeks passed, and Dr. D'Adamo called me. This is how that chat went:

"Hi Allan, it's Dr. D'Adamo. . . ."

(Deep breath . . . followed by my very pregnant pause)

"Hello? Allan, are you there?"

"Yes, hi, Dr. D'Adamo. How are you? I really can't talk now, I'm late for a class—"

"I'll just be a moment, Allan. . . ."

Fat chance.

He went on to explain that he was working on a new book and that he had tried collaborating with other writers, but they didn't work out. He said he felt there had been a good flow between us with the first book and hoped we could team up again.

I was flattered, I told him. But didn't he say everything that he wanted to say in *One Man's Food*? And what about Peter's books? They were international bestsellers. Why do another book? Didn't he capture it all? Anyway, I was very busy. I hoped he would understand that I wasn't interested.

But it was as if he hadn't heard a word I said. "I've been practicing for 50 years now, Allan, and have treated 50,000-plus patients. I've made new discoveries . . . there are sub–blood types . . . and no, Peter's book isn't the final word on this. I don't agree with his idea of lectins. And I'm still trying to heal people one by one; he's trying to heal the world through the Internet. Besides, I was wrong about certain things. . . ."

My first thought was that there was a father-son competition going on. The father, who is the founding father of blood groups and the godfather of naturopathic doctors in the United States, may have wanted the last word on his own discovery.

But what did he mean he was wrong about certain things? It isn't typical for doctors to admit mistakes. I had never doubted Dr. D'Adamo's ethics; he was a purist compared to the many practitioners I had met in the '80s, when the alternative-health movement exploded in the U.S. So I took it seriously when he said that he had made mistakes and the blood-type groups might not be what he originally said they were. But that didn't mean I wanted to write a second book with him.

"I'd like to talk more, but I have to give my students a final—"

"Think it over, Allan."

He asked for my address so he could send me material on his work to help me think it over.

Fifty years of research and 50,000-plus patients echoed in my mind as I caught the elevator up to my classroom. *Three decades hadn't dampened his passion for his work,* I mused. His voice still had the same commanding power it had 30 years ago. I thought about the first time he asked me to work with him. It was about six weeks after I had become his patient. He looked at me and said, "You are going to write my book."

But that was then. I was younger, hungrier for an assignment. I had no children, fewer obligations . . . and I didn't supervise a journalism–mass communication program with students and faculty alike knocking at my door all day long.

Reunion

So why am I now in a hotel in Portsmouth, New Hampshire, late in the evening, writing these notes for the Introduction to his book? I suppose I came here out of curiosity. We were the co-authors of a book that launched a worldwide movement in blood types and diet, and while I've been far removed from that world for three decades, I thought that Dr. D'Adamo is such an original thinker and naturopath that I should at least hear what he had to say.

The doctor and his wife, Christiana, picked me up at Manchester-Boston Regional Airport two days ago. I've spent the time touring his institute (two joined New England–style wood-frame houses in downtown Portsmouth) and being introduced to his staff of trained naturopaths and an array of therapies, including German footbaths, a hyperbaric chamber, and a Firard sauna he added to his trade over the years and used for treating cancer, rheumatoid arthritis, and arteriosclerosis. After work hours we walked the wooded grounds of his 17-acre farm, stopping first at a meditation area replete with a Buddha and bench by a stream, and then at a gazebo near his herb garden, where we reconnected first as men and later as professionals.

I commented that this was a far cry from the backyard of his home in Staten Island where I interviewed him for our first book. "Even further from my childhood . . ." he said. He was alluding to his life as the son of a beat cop who pounded the pavement in some of the toughest areas of New York City.

But Dr. D'Adamo wasn't interested in reflecting. He was as passionate about his work as ever, and I had to pull in the reins a number of times when he was ready to go on about blood types and his newest observations: about why a B, such as me, should avoid soy milk and limit consumption of chicken; and then particularly about sub–blood groups, A1's and H1's, and the impact of Rh factors.

It seemed he had a storehouse of new information and was eager for me to turn on my tape recorder so I could document it all. I was interested in hearing what he had to say, but I was more content, at first, to study and reacquaint myself with him.

I asked him what he thought about integrative medicine, the movement of medical doctors like Andrew Weil who are merging traditional medicine with alternative medicine. That sparked an immediate and fiery response. He waved his hand emphatically, like a prophet of discontent.

"What do the medical doctors know about naturopathic medicine—for years so many medical doctors denounced naturopathic techniques, and now they want to practice it. If they want to practice, let them get the appropriate training. Have they studied and practiced using botanicals or acupuncture? Many are dabbling, jumping on a bandwagon of alternative medicine, which is enormous in America because so many people are dissatisfied with the medical profession."

This was prime D'Adamo. He was still breathing fire when it came to defending the naturopathic approach. He also had a historic vantage point—he had spent 50 years treating patients based on the blood-type approach. What other American naturopathic doctor had his experience?

I probed further, asking him how he felt now that so many Americans had become more involved with alternative-healing methods. I noted that America was not like this when we wrote our first book. People who followed a natural lifestyle and alternative-health practitioners were considered faddists, even quacks.

Today, many people commonly eat organic foods, practice yoga, see acupuncturists, and take vitamins and herbs. The alternative-health movement—and the concept of preventive medicine—is much more widespread.

"Yes, it's wonderful to see people become more conscious of things like yoga and meditation and vitamins and diet," he replied. "You used to need a doctor's prescription to buy raw milk from a health-food store in New York, if you could even find one in New York 30 to 40 years ago. Can you imagine that? Now you can buy organic milk in the local supermarket. But developing the awareness is only step one. Individuals still need to know whether raw milk is good for their bodies, or whether they need to do a calming exercise like yoga or more rigorous ones like running or swimming. Or whether they should eat lamb or organ meats, or be a vegetarian.

"On top of that, there are so many so-called healthy superfood combinations being popularized on the Internet to increase energy or for infertility or weight reduction—they're not only preposterous, they can be outright harmful. Recommending concentrated mixed-juice diets, which are loaded with sugar, as a quick pick-me-up to people who are chronically fatigued could take them down the road to hypoglycemia or even diabetes, if they aren't already there. It still comes back to knowing what foods are right for an individual based on blood type and current state of health."

Second Time Around

That last comment was the reason I decided to collaborate with Dr. D'Adamo again. Here was the naturopathic doctor who had arguably made the most original contribution to natural healing in modern times, with 30 *more* years of experience in treating disease. This, at a time when Americans are more willing than ever to take responsibility for their health and explore new paths to healing. It seemed like a propitious moment for us to work together again.

It's now 3 A.M. in Portsmouth. Tomorrow morning, I will turn on the tape recorder and start capturing what Dr. D'Adamo has been yearning to reveal: his latest observations and discoveries about blood type and healing, and how he addresses some of the most challenging diseases of the 21st century, including obesity, heart disease, cancer, diabetes, ADD, and depression. And more, he shares his urgent new message about prevention—something sorely missing from the American health-care movement. The rest, for me, will be in the telling.

— Allan Richards
Portsmouth, New Hampshire

CHAPTER ONE

The Original Blood-Type Diet

In my first book, *One Man's Food . . . is someone else's poison,* published in 1980, I (Dr. James D'Adamo) set out to do two things: stake a claim for the naturopathic approach to healing in the United States; and reveal for the first time my discovery of the correlation between a person's blood type and his or her diet as a means of maximizing health, as well as a method of treating diseases, even the leading causes of death in the United States—heart disease, cancer, diabetes, and chronic obstructive pulmonary disease (COPD).

In my second book, *The D'Adamo Diet,* which I wrote in 1989, I described my discoveries about sub–blood groups and Rh factors, and their impact on individualized diets.

Much has been written based on my work on blood types since *One Man's Food* first appeared, including *The New York Times* bestseller *Eat Right 4 Your Type* by my son Dr. Peter D'Adamo, who is also a naturopath. While I'm gratified that many health practitioners have shown an interest in my research and work, and in Peter's case, shared my concept of blood types with millions of readers around the world, it's also disappointing to see how many nutritionists have latched onto the blood-type concept as if it were the latest fad and incorporated the basis of my discoveries into their practice or publications without having actually treated a significant number of patients.

Blood Type and the Individual

One Man's Food not only launched the idea of a correlation between a person's blood and diet, but also espoused a radical idea—*radical* when compared to the way most medical doctors, and even some nutritionists, practice today: that each person is a unique creation with specific characteristics. In other words, there are no two people on the face of the earth who are alike—no two people have the same fingerprints, lip prints, ear lobes, irises, or voices (identical twins don't even share all of the same characteristics); therefore, no two people should eat the same foods.

Blood type is a highly popular concept now—it even has its proponents who say that blood type defines personality. Its significance as a nutritional tool is one I have pioneered and developed over a period of 50 years. Its new marketability, although welcome, as this means reaching a wider audience, exposes it to practitioners who benefit from association with the concept but lack substantive knowledge or application of it.

At the time I wrote *One Man's Food,* I had examined, diagnosed, and treated more than 15,000 patients. I had a successful practice in Bay Ridge, Brooklyn, a quiet Italian community just inland from the towering Verrazano-Narrows Bridge, which connects Brooklyn to Staten Island; an office on the Upper West Side of Manhattan; and another office on Hester Street in Little Italy where I treated the poor. It's a time I think of as the end of the Dark Ages of natural healing in the United States. The American naturopathic movement—the natural approach to health—was only then beginning to emerge from the underground into the mainstream.

Fast Forward

Although naturopathy in this country dates back to the late 1800s and saw various spikes in popularity in the 1920s and '30s, it started to find a broader audience during the 1960s, when many traditional approaches to life—including conventional medicine, which treats symptoms, not causes, and essentially views all people as having the same type of body—were being challenged.

The baby-boomer generation sought alternatives to many aspects of modern society—a society that had become more and more mechanistic and had increasingly removed itself from nature. The concern we see today for climate change and global warming isn't new. The environmental movement and the quest for cleaner air and purer water and foods (that weren't colored and preserved with artificial ingredients, including some identified as cancer-causing agents) was a response to a world that had relied on pesticides to produce vegetables and fruits; antibiotics and hormones to fatten beef and chicken; and whose industries and vehicles produced massive amounts of carbon dioxide and other pollutants that clouded our cities and increased the incidence of asthma and other respiratory conditions.

The lay public and scientists alike began to recognize that our way of life was choking us; and that obesity, heart disease, and other chronic diseases particular to industrialized society were fostered by the daily consumption of processed foods.

In many ways, America was far behind European nations like Germany and Switzerland, which were much more conscientious about safeguarding their foodstuffs—their organically grown tomatoes, green vegetables, grapes, cherries, and other fruits weren't pale and tasteless imitations of the real things, as they so often are in this country. In addition, ailments were commonly treated with therapies that we call alternative—*alternative* meaning to us another approach to the medical doctor's five-minute diagnosis and prescribing of pharmaceuticals. Physicians in European countries employed herbs and botanicals, homeopathic remedies, water and mineral therapies, and many other gentle and effective remedies drawn from nature.

Young people in America began to experiment with vegetarianism, macrobiotics, and natural therapies, and advanced the idea that *we* are responsible for our own well-being and could take preventive steps to secure the great gift of health. This wasn't something the American Medical Association or the pharmaceutical companies cheerfully encouraged because health care in this country was then, and still is, about profit—more specifically, profit from people's illnesses. Michael Moore's 2007 documentary *SiCKO* is an accurate portrayal of the American health-care system: if you can't pay for it, suffer.

It has never been easy being a naturopathic doctor in this country, or again, what's referred to as an "alternative practitioner" in America, advocating the use of food or herbs as medicine for prevention or to help heal disease. When I started practicing in the 1950s, I couldn't even suggest, as I do today, that I could help patients suffering with cancer overcome it through diet—even though it's largely a food-associated disease.

If news that food is medicine was newly bursting on the American health scene in the 1960s, my concept of blood types and the idea that people should be treated as individuals, one by one, and not as carbon copies of each other, was also a fresh idea, although conventional-minded people often thought of it as a half-baked premise. And yet, as I based my treatments on the correlation between blood types and diet and helped bring relief to my patients, word spread around New York City and beyond about my discovery and approach; and my offices overflowed with people, many suffering with advanced states of diseases.

American Health Care: The Need for Prevention

Today, three decades later, there is a different climate in terms of health care in America. However, the American health system is deeply troubled. Chronic diseases such as heart disease, cancer, diabetes, and obesity account for more than 70 percent of U.S. health-care costs, according to the Centers for Disease Control and Prevention (CDC). Yet those who suffer from these diseases receive only about 50 percent of the recommended preventive care. One out of every four deaths in the United States is due to cancer. Over 65 percent of Americans are overweight; and the CDC estimates that obesity causes more than 112,000 deaths a year and is at the root of other conditions including diabetes, hypertension, arthritis, respiratory problems, depression, and gynecological complications, including infertility.

Yet I believe—I *know*—that cancer and these chronic conditions are preventable, and if these diseases were prevented or treated using my research and work in blood types, we could save well over $100 billion a year in health-care spending.

Today the powerful pharmaceutical companies still manage to get their drugs to the marketplace—many that have long lists of serious side effects or have not been tested long enough and are harmful to the body. (For example, Vioxx, a medication for arthritis, led to approximately 30,000 cardiac deaths before it was pulled from the market in 2004.)

Fortunately, there's also a greater awareness of the role food plays in healing.

When I moved to Portsmouth, New Hampshire, 10 years ago, after practicing in my institutes in Brooklyn and Toronto and an office in Montreal for 40 years, I sought to wind down my practice and devote more time to teaching my work on blood types to other naturopaths. And yet the patients kept coming to see me: patients from as far away as California, Hong Kong, the Philippines, Mexico, and South America; patients from countries with socialized medicine, like England and France; and even patients who had health insurance and could afford expensive conventional medical treatments (few of my treatments are covered by insurance). Why would they do this? Why would they spend thousands of dollars and travel halfway around the world for the individualized programs that I created for them? Because what my father told me as a boy is true: good health is a person's greatest treasure, and there's not much you can do without it.

I'm gratified to see the growing awareness people have about the importance of foods, herbs, and exercise with respect to their health. Many medical doctors still label alternative approaches to healing—even mine—as "quackery" because proof of their effectiveness and the way the techniques work haven't been scientifically verified, although the results can certainly be observed. Yet they nevertheless have had to start incorporating natural remedies into their practice because millions of Americans are using them and enjoying their benefits.

Yet this heightened awareness is only one step in the prevention and treatment of chronic disease. My clarion call after practicing for 50 years and treating over 50,000 patients is the same: all people are unique individuals, created by the shared genetics of two parents; molded by their culture, society, and geographic region in which they were raised and live; and directed by their dominant thoughts.

Most important, a person's blood type—whether it is O, A, B, or AB—is nature's most reliable guide in determining their individualized dietary needs.

I want to qualify this statement, and that's the reason I decided to write *Maximise Your Health with the Blood Type Diet.* In the years since *One Man's Food* was published, I've continued to research the nature of blood types and discovered that there is even more to creating individualized diets than the correlation between food and the four types of blood. My additional research has confirmed the significance of sub–blood groups, which appear in individuals whose parents and grandparents have different blood types. For instance, an individual who is Type O may have underlying characteristics of A or B, while an A may have several traits of an O or a B.

Moreover, I've similarly discovered that Rh factors (Rh-positive and Rh-negative) and A1's and H1's, other qualities of the blood that can be determined through serum typing, also play a role in creating a person's individual diet and treatment. People who are Rh-positive tend to respond more readily to the blood-type program; Rh-negative people, I have found, respond slowly to treatment. Type O's who are H1 positive require more protein than O's who are H1-negative type. Type A's who are A1 positive require protein with a vegetarian diet; A's who are A1 negative require less protein or can be total vegetarians.

As you can see, blood typing is complex, and there's much more to it than just a general understanding of the four blood groups. Through years of research and working with the blood's various qualities, I've been able to achieve greater and more dramatic success in healing the most debilitating diseases of our time.

This book is the sum of my years employing my system of healing, and provides the latest information about blood types and diet, which you can follow to improve your general health. But it also poses a challenge to the medical profession and those who claim to be blood-type-diet practitioners by revealing how my expanded work in blood types can prevent as well as heal chronic diseases—cancer, heart disease, diabetes, obesity, hypoglycemia, and depression . . . diseases that continue to bankrupt the nation's health-care system and needlessly cause human suffering.

CHAPTER TWO

Blood Types and Prevention

Two of the most memorable case histories in my years of treating patients involve two young boys. In the first case, the boy, Roger, suffered with attention deficit disorder (ADD). It's fairly normal for boys of nine to be highly energetic and active, and Roger was no different—he was in a state of perpetual motion. However, there is a qualitative difference between being active and being frenetic. Like many children who have ADD, Roger couldn't sit still or focus his mind for a prolonged period. At school, he was disruptive in the classroom, frequently shouting out during the teacher's lesson or arguing with his classmates during recess, which often led to fights.

Roger had been treated by medical doctors and received the typical battery of medications, such as Ritalin, but with limited results. His parents brought him to me in my Toronto clinic as a last resort—many patients find their way into my office after they've gone the route of conventional medicine without finding much success. And conventional medicine had failed Roger bigtime—his mother grew hysterical as she explained that he had set their house on fire.

I had no easy answer for the parents when they asked, "Why did our son burn down the house?" There could have been any number of reasons for Roger's emotional and psychological state and his extreme actions, but I didn't want to speculate. But this I knew implicitly: many conditions, including ADD, are a result of an imbalance in the body's biochemistry and can be treated nutritionally and through vitamin supplementation. I explained that I work from the inside out and try to restore order to the body using nutrition, based on a person's blood type. If they were willing to trust me and follow my recommendations—in Roger's case to the maximum—we might be able to normalize his behavior.

Roger's father said he'd read about the correlation of blood type and genetics in the Pulitzer prize–winning book *Guns, Germs, and Steel: The Fates of Human Societies* by Jared Diamond, an evolutionary scientist and professor of geography and physiology at UCLA. He later brought in the book and shared the following quotation, which describes a person's resistance to disease based on blood groups:

> . . . the differential mortality from epidemic diseases in traditional European societies had little to do with intelligence, and instead involved genetic resistance dependent on details of body chemistry. For example, people with blood group B or O have a greater resistance to smallpox than do people with blood group A.

The fact that he had read something pertaining to blood types and disease probably reduced his skepticism that ADD could be treated by adjusting his son's diet according to his type of blood. His wife was less given to intellectualizing about whether my approach was scientifically based. I am known in Toronto for having success with a number of conditions through nutrition and various supplements—ADD is one of them—and she went full steam ahead with the program.

ADD: An Inner Tsunami

Roger was a Type O. I will more fully explain the O's physical and emotional qualities and dietary needs later, but generally speaking, the O has a robust and active nature and needs daily helpings of animal protein. I recommended that Roger follow a high-protein diet, starting with a protein shake upon rising before breakfast; and then eating an assortment of seven small servings of fish, meat, turkey, buffalo, and/or lamb at two-hour intervals throughout the day.

I also greatly reduced his intake of carbohydrates—breads, pasta, and mashed potatoes, all of which, when digested, break down into glucose; and I immediately eliminated all sources of sugar from his diet including honey, candy bars, soft drinks, fruit juices, maple syrup (which Roger used in generous helpings on his pancakes on a daily basis), and any foods sweetened with high-fructose corn syrup (which also breaks down into pure glucose when digested).

It is now common knowledge—you can even see advertisements for high-energy drinks on television that refer to this—that sugar in any form, including fruit sugars, jolts the body with a wave of energy. To a boy with ADD or a disposition to hyperactivity, the ongoing jolts produce a chaotic, surging force. I liken it to a stormy internal sea. Imagine watching waves crashing into a shoreline or rocky coast. Sugar agitates and stirs the bloodstream with that same kind of wild energy. The forces raging inside Roger must have had the power of an inner tsunami in order to provoke him to set fire to his family home.

Although it might not seem so, a body that is subjected to ongoing surges and is in constant motion is actually very tired and depleted. The constant intake of protein would supply slowly digested nourishment that, with the reduction of carbohydrates and sugar, would help even out Roger's blood-sugar level, restore and rebuild his strength, and allow his body to find its inherent energy. A daily regimen of B vitamins, of doses specific to his condition and blood type, was also vital to nourishing and soothing his nervous system.

Roger responded to the diet fairly quickly and gained enough control over his emotional and psychological states so that within several months he was able to return to school where, for the first time, he started to excel.

Asthma and Diet

The second boy, Ivan, is an example of the impact of irresponsible parenting on a child's health. Ivan suffered with severe asthma and frequently visited the ER, wheezing, coughing, and gasping for air. He had Type A blood. A's are highly sensitive to dairy products—a small glass of milk, a slice of cheese, or a scoop of ice cream is like poison to their bodies. Ivan's body reacted by producing an excessive amount of mucous plugs that clogged his airways.

I immediately eliminated all dairy foods, then wheat products, which are far too acidic for an A, and placed him on a strict vegetarian diet. The A is the only blood type that should be 100 percent vegetarian, although in some cases there may be traits of other blood types that can modify an A's needs.

Within weeks of following my recommendations, Ivan's lungs cleared of the congestion, and he was able to stop using his steroid inhaler. He resumed a normal life, which included daily sports activities at school.

About two months later, however, Ivan was back in my office wheezing wildly. I suspected that he had gone off his diet and was again eating dairy products. Ivan's mother confided in me that he often watched TV and ate ice cream and cookies at night when his father came home from work.

I rarely lose my temper with a patient, but I took Ivan's father into the hall outside my office and read him the riot act. I told him that if he wanted to eat ice cream and cookies that was *his* business, but why destroy his son's chance at a healthy life? Ivan's mother made sure there were no more desserts in front of the TV set. Ivan's asthmatic reactions again receded.

Prevention Tips?

I often think of Roger and Ivan and how their lives dramatically changed upon following the appropriate diet for their blood types. I had them—and many other patients—in mind a lot during the 2008 political campaign because downtown Portsmouth, where my institute is located, was one of the first stops on the primary trail and all through the presidential campaign, candidates of every stripe flocked here trying to sell their programs.

Health care again emerged as a major issue, and though some politicians like to refer to the United States' health-care system as the "best in the world," it was rated last or next to last in terms of quality by the prestigious Commonwealth Fund when compared with Australia, Canada, Germany, New Zealand, and the United Kingdom.

While I support universal health insurance, I also fervently believe that even if we modify our approach to health care, many millions of Americans will still suffer needlessly. We're ignoring the most important part of health care: *prevention.*

Our health-care system is backward. We try to treat a condition once it's firmly established in the body, but we spend little time or money in educating the public about the importance of the food they put into their bodies and how to prevent conditions from developing in the first place.

In a recent report by the Partnership for Prevention, a non-profit health-policy group, health experts, including doctors for the CDC, said that increased use of just five preventive services would save more than 100,000 lives every year in the United States. "This shows so dramatically the potential impact of prevention," said Dr. Kathleen Toomey of the CDC, which helped fund the study. "Our nation has never truly invested in prevention."

The catch, even in this report, are the five recommended prevention tips. Let me review them for you:

1. Take a low-dose aspirin every day to prevent heart disease.

2. Have regular screenings for colorectal cancer.

3. Have regular breast-cancer screenings.

4. Quit smoking.

5. Get annual flu shots if you are over 50.

Of course, people shouldn't smoke and should have periodic screenings for cancer, but the basis of prevention—the importance of our daily foods—is absent from this list. If we're referring to food-associated diseases, how can we have a health-care system that fails to stress the impact of the food that we put into our bodies?

Scientists have long had ample evidence about the correlation between certain foods and chronic disease. The National Research Council, for example, cited massive evidence in a report called "Diet, Nutrition and Cancer" in 1982, linking dietary factors to breast cancer.

Even the U.S. Department of Health and Human Services (HHS) and the U.S. Department of Agriculture (USDA) provide science-based advice to promote health and reduce risk for chronic diseases through diet and physical activity in the 2005 *Dietary Guidelines for Americans*:

> Good nutrition is vital to good health and is absolutely essential for the healthy growth and development of children and adolescents. . . . Specific diseases and conditions linked to poor diet include cardiovascular disease, hypertension, dyslipidemia, type 2 diabetes, overweight and obesity, osteoporosis, constipation, diverticular disease, iron deficiency anemia, oral disease, malnutrition, and some cancers.

Understanding Food

Today, modern medical doctors are gradually finding their way back to what Hippocrates proclaimed 2,500 years ago: "Let thy foods be thy medicine and thy medicine thy food." They increasingly offer what they think are sound nutritional ideas in magazine articles or postings on Websites. But what are these mainstream practitioners recommending?

Eat beetroot, they say, because beetroot are a good source of folate and betaine, two nutrients that help lower blood levels of homocysteine, a compound that can damage arteries and increase your risk of heart disease. Or drink pomegranate juice because taken over a year it can reduce blood pressure. Or eat tomatoes because they contain lycopene, which fights cancer.

Yet these recommendations and many others are general comments. Beetroot and pomegranate juice—and carrot juice, another popular health drink—also have high levels of glucose (sugar), which, if you have hypoglycemia or low blood sugar, would only further stress your pancreas and adrenal glands and heighten your fatigue. If Roger had been drinking carrot or pomegranate juice on a regular basis, he would never have come to grips with ADD and his frenetic behavior.

And those poor people who are trying to get the protective benefits of lycopene from tomatoes, tomato sauce, or ketchup would have to eat a couple hundred tomatoes per week! Even if they have the time and wherewithal to eat so many tomatoes, that amount would be far too acidic for most people, especially for those with gastric conditions or Type B blood.

The heart of my belief and practice, as I've said—although it can never be said too often—is that every individual is a unique creation composed of two different sets of genetic traits that come together only once in this universe, and never again. I believe there are no human stereotypes, no carbon copies, no perfect replications—similarities, yes, relatedness, definitely; but even members of the same family have vast differences among them. And subsequently, no two people can eat the same two diets.

Early in my career, my studies in blood pathology led me to explore the possibility of a link between an individual's blood quality and the body's characteristics, including the person's dietary needs. Further, my observation about blood types and sub–blood groups and the importance of eating wisely, with the knowledge of which foods give strength to the individual body (and not according to the iron rule of your taste buds), has healed the infirm; but perhaps just as significant, it has also prevented chronic illness in many.

The same way in which a medical doctor writes prescriptions for drugs to fight symptoms, I write menus, recommending (as needed) particular fruits, vegetables, animal proteins, and grains specific to an individual's blood type, sub–blood type, and the current physical condition of his or her body. The same way in which most people take a drug to relieve them of a symptom, my patients use food to strengthen and balance their bodies and help protect them from losing their natural vitality; and in the case of a disease, heal the root cause of the problem. So yes, I might recommend beetroot, pomegranate, or carrot juice; or okra, brown rice, or any number of foods, but it's according to the patient's individual needs.

Avoiding Disease

Not long ago, I read an article in *The Boston Globe* about a former patient of mine who was running in the Boston Marathon. I was gratified because only three years ago, this woman was struggling with breast cancer. While I'm always excited about being able to help patients regain their health, as I was with this woman, I also know that if she had only understood which foods she needed to eat *before* her body was compromised, before she developed the cancer, it could have been prevented.

The cancer victim, the diabetic, the infertile woman, the child with ADD, the depressed teenager, the prematurely crippled arthritic . . . all of the many beautiful lovers of life who hunger for health, the many who are cut down before they should have been, not by war or because they were impoverished and couldn't afford a bag of groceries, but because of a bag filled with the absolutely wrong food for their blood types—none of them should have ever suffered so.

While politicians try to find a cure for the ailing health-care system in the United States, you and your family can quietly partake in a real health-care revolution by treating yourself as individuals and *preventing* the chronic illnesses that continue to strike so many.

CHAPTER THREE

Blood Types: Truth of Nature

Every day, all around the world, people watch plasma-screen televisions, talk on cell phones that take photographs and broadcast news, and drive self-parking cars. All of these wonders of the 21st century rely on sophisticated technologies and come with operating manuals.

Our complex physical, emotional, psychological, and spiritual bodies are increasingly read through our individual DNA . . . but our stories are also written in our blood.

By deciphering the qualities inherent in the different blood types (O, A, B, or AB), I have been able to guide thousands of people around the world to a better understanding of their nutritional needs.

The people who use this information rise to the level of health that nature intended for their unique bodies, while at the same time helping to prevent the most common degenerative diseases.

Again, let me acknowledge that many of us are already on a better path of health than those of previous generations. We buy foods made of organically grown ingredients and eat produce from local family farms. Community-supported agriculture programs and farmers' markets—even in urban areas like New York City and Boston—offer consumers access to vegetables, meats, and grains that are fresher and significantly more nutritious than food shipped across the country (most of America's food is picked four to seven days before being shipped on average a thousand miles to market, including health-food stores).

Today, almost five million American adults are practicing vegetarians, and 25 percent of the entire American population are "flexitarians," according to the American Dietetic Association. Flexitarians eat a mostly plant-based diet composed of grains, vegetables, and fruits but also include dairy or lean meat, such as buffalo, fish, poultry, or ostrich two or three days a week.

Just about everyone in America is experimenting with one kind of diet or other. Still, with food-associated diseases like obesity and cancer claiming more than a half-million lives a year, we do need to pay more attention to our dietary habits. But what kind of diet?

When I talk about a blood-type diet, I'm not referring to a faddish regimen or a weight-reduction program. I'm talking about what I believe—and have proved time and time again—is a Truth in nature. I'm talking about understanding your individual makeup and the foods that are appropriate for your body.

So if you have Type A blood and are one of those five million Americans who are following a vegetarian diet, I would say you're probably on a good track. However, if you're a Type O, which is a very physically active type that requires a daily diet of animal protein, you're depriving your body of much-needed nutrition. In time you'll diminish your body's inherent vitality, experience fatigue and lassitude, and render yourself vulnerable to disease.

But that doesn't have to happen to the O or anyone—provided you follow the path defined by your blood type.

Type O

Let's take a closer look at Type O and determine why that person should be following a high-protein diet.

Over 50 percent of all my patients are O's. The O is constitutionally the strongest of all the blood types and has the longest life expectancy. Type O usually has a well-developed physique and thrives on physical activity. O's, in fact, are the athletes of the world. Although they tend to be muscular, their blood flow can be sluggish, and without a vigorous exercise program of an hour or more per day to stimulate the circulatory system, they (more than any of the other blood types) will rapidly grow lethargic. Through vigorous physical exercise, people who are Type O not only recharge their batteries and optimize their physical energy, but they also gain the kind of mental clarity needed by high achievers.

This takes us back to the O's need for animal protein.

If we return to an earlier period of humankind's development, we will note, as the anthropologists tell us—and was also described in my son Peter's book *Eat Right 4 Your Type*—that the first blood type to appear was an O. Early man was a hunter, dependent on physical prowess to track and kill his food. The fight-or-flight syndrome was also never called upon more than in our ancestors whose daily survival was exceedingly tenuous. That man required high-octane fuel, and that fuel came from his regular consumption of the most energy-packed food substance: animal protein.

Although few of us today hunt for our next meal, and our fight-or-flight mechanism is triggered far less than in other periods of human history, Type O's still bear the imprint of their predecessors and require daily helpings of animal protein to meet their physical needs.

An O who tries to lead a vegetarian lifestyle will always be hungry and constantly snacking—usually on a carbohydrate—to get a quick boost. O's who follow this regimen will ultimately develop hypoglycemia, or low blood sugar. Hypoglycemia strikes roughly 65 to 85 percent of all Americans and results from the intake of an excessive amount of sugar from carbohydrates and alcohol (as well as too many cups of coffee or caffeinated herbal energy drinks), which causes the pancreas to oversecrete insulin.

All carbohydrates—including root vegetables, fruits, and grains, as well as cane or brown sugar—break down into glucose when digested. The pancreas secretes insulin into the blood to reg-ulate the glucose, but in a hypoglycemic person, too much insulin is released and blood sugar quickly drops to unhealthy levels.

All cells of the body take up glucose for fuel, but when the glu-cose level is too low, the cells hunger for fuel, often causing physi-cal, mental, and emotional fatigue. Untreated, hypoglycemia can eventually produce a host of diseases from depression to diabetes and cancer.

Hypoglycemia is more commonly found in an O who's deprived of animal protein than in any other blood type.

For optimal health, O's should include several servings of tur-key, lamb, fish, and occasionally organic beef in their daily diet. However, an O should limit or entirely eliminate dairy and wheat products. Milk, cheese, and eggs produce an excessive amount of mucus in the O, which often leads to chronic respiratory and circu-latory conditions. Type O's who eliminate or greatly reduce dairy products from their diet will prevent or dramatically improve their asthma or chronic sinus conditions.

Of all the blood types, O's naturally tend to suffer the fewest circulatory and cardiac-related diseases. But an O who consumes dairy products on a regular basis will respond more like an A—the A's develop the greatest number of heart-related diseases of all the blood types—and develop excessive plaque in their arteries, lead-ing to any number of circulatory and cardiac diseases.

Wheat products are similarly disruptive to an O's body and can create an imbalance of hydrochloric acid in the O's stomach. So they're no strangers to antacid tablets, as they naturally have hyperacidity of the stomach. Upsetting the acid level makes the O susceptible to a number of digestive and abdominal conditions including duodenal ulcers, gastritis, and acid reflux. As you can see, even when you try to follow what you believe is a healthy diet (aren't we told that whole-wheat bread is healthier than white-bread products?), you can still be choosing the wrong foods for your body.

But the key to health for O's isn't just in the foods they select. A preventive lifestyle must include vigorous exercise. Remember, the O was a hunter. So whether you're a student listening to lectures all day, a high-powered account executive, or a salesperson, if you are an O, you need rigorous cardiovascular exercise such as jogging, gymnastics, calisthenics, hiking, swimming, or bicycling.

Type O's who eat protein but don't exercise turn the positive effects and health benefits of the protein into a toxic situation for their bodies. They'll struggle with rapid weight gain and battle bulges, double chins, and a growing lassitude until they resume a fitness regime.

Exercising at the appropriate time is also imperative. The best time for an O to work out is first thing in the morning. Those who do so invigorate their entire system and create a barrier against stress and anxiety. O's who exercise in the evening will receive the cardiovascular benefits but not the same mental and emotional benefits.

Please note: For Type O's who are ill or incapacitated, they must reduce protein intake and exercise only to their capacity.

Type A

The optimal preventive diet for an A is, as I previously noted, vegetarian based. Whereas the O's were nomadic hunters and cave dwellers, the A's developed during a time when people created settlements and turned to farming. Lifestyle changes led to nutritional changes. You can appreciate this better by thinking about your daily life. If you work all day in an office, are a suburbanite who drives more than you walk, or if you spend too much time in front of the television or on the Internet, you don't have the same need for large protein-based meals as someone who has a more physically demanding occupation, such as a farmer, a forest ranger, or a plumber.

So as people organized into societies, they relied more on their intellect than on their physical strength alone, and a new blood type emerged. More than 35 percent of my patients are A's.

A's, in general, are less active than O's, and their bodies don't have the same need for animal protein. Unlike the O's body, which is predisposed toward hyperacidity, A's lack sufficient hydrochloric

acid in the stomach, which makes the digestion of protein difficult for them. In fact, no matter how well Type A individuals eat
or how many vitamins they take, their bodies are still unable to
completely break down and assimilate food or supplements, so
it's necessary for them to take hydrochloric betaine supplements
and rennet tablets to help digest their food. (Rennet is commonly
used in making cheese, as it causes the protein in milk to curdle
and is generally obtained from the stomach lining of young milk-
fed calves or goats, although there are non-animal sources suitable
for vegetarian consumption. In combination with hydrochloric
betaine supplements, rennet accelerates the breaking down of
mucus.)

Because Type A's typically suffer from mucous-related conditions and frequently experience colds, sinus infections, allergies,
and other respiratory problems, they must avoid dairy products.
Any dairy—a drop of milk or a slice of cheese—in an A's body is
absolute poison. The only milk an A can tolerate and digest is
breast milk at infancy.

In addition, an A should avoid whole-wheat products (although
an A can tolerate germinated wheat, as the acid is neutralized). The
most beneficial foods to the A will always be those that are more
alkaline-forming, including leafy green vegetables, tofu, soy milk,
and an assortment of grains like rice, quinoa, spelt, amaranth, and
rice- or soy-based pastas.

As I noted, A's developed an acute intellect as they adapted to
a community-oriented lifestyle and are known for their strong rea-
soning powers. They are the problem solvers. Nothing is too complex for the A to work through. Likewise, because they're acutely
sensitive, A's are more closely connected to their emotional nature
and are highly creative. They tend to be interested in culture and
the arts; and because they're deeply spiritual, their artistic pursuits
often have a transcendent quality, with frequent references to the
divine. I would speculate here that artists such as Michelangelo or
the poet Percy Bysshe Shelley, who was a vegetarian, were Type A's.

They also tend to have overstimulated minds, which heighten
their metabolic rates. For all their intellectual, artistic, and spiritual depth, those who are Type A are driven by nervous kinetic

energy and rarely experience their true natural energy. They're always on the go—mentally, physically, and emotionally. On the surface, it's easy to confuse an A for an O because they both seem active and vital. But the A is at the mercy of a restless mind, not a body yearning for movement.

This kind of erratic energy produces internal tension, turmoil, and impatience. Type A's will frequently start a project or school-work, only to leave it unfinished. They may feel the need to travel or escape their circumstances. Stressed and nervous, they can be hypercritical of themselves and others, and difficult to please.

Because of the A's intellectual capacity and kinetic drive, they appear to be good multitaskers. Again, however, these individuals mistake their multitasking skills as a sign of physical strength. Their perpetual motion eventually catches up with them as it wears down their pancreas, adrenals, and heart, as well as triggering premature aging. It's as if they use up their body's supply of vital energy and are suddenly old. Because of this, Type A individuals have the shortest life expectancy of all the blood types, although they can add useful years by eating and exercising appropriately based on their blood group.

Developing an inner calm is, therefore, one of the keys to the A's health and prevention program. They need to live in a serene environment and aren't the type of people who will tolerate living in an apartment in midtown Manhattan, with blaring car horns and endless bustle. They'll often find themselves looking for a patch of green under a quiet tree in Central Park and will have many sleepless nights until they move to a calmer setting.

Exercise is as important to the A as it is to the O, but the A's workout must be oriented toward soothing the body, not further exciting it. Activities such as jogging, calisthenics, gymnastics, or contact sports will have a stimulating effect on the nervous system and further agitate an A. Those who are Type A should practice yoga, tai chi, or qi gong, which will help elongate rigid muscles and release stored tension. Practicing yoga upon rising will help center and prepare A's for the day. For those who have difficulty sleeping, I recommend that they remain in a lotus position after completing their *asanas* (yogic postures) and repeat the word *peace* as a mantra. Words affect internal states, and this will help soothe the mind.

Meditation, too, will help center Type A individuals and encourage a sense of peace, especially if practiced first thing in the morning. They may find it difficult to turn off their active minds, but they can learn to harness their mental energy as they develop a daily discipline. Five-minute meditation breaks every few hours will keep their minds quiet and focused, and also have a rejuvenating effect.

Try the following simple exercise before going to sleep: Lie down on your bed or a flat mat on the floor, take a few gentle breaths, and focus on your muscles and inner organs. Tune in to your inner tensions. You'll be amazed that five to ten minutes of relaxation can release tight muscles, especially around the upper shoulders and neck area.

This simple exercise can help you identify the impact that thoughts have on your body—that is, which thoughts drain your energy, and which fill you with a sense of serenity and well-being.

Type B

We all know the expression "Everything in moderation." No blood type epitomizes the middle way more than a B. The preventive diet and exercise regimen for a Type B falls right in between the O and the A. When in a balanced state of health, a B requires the best of both kingdoms: animal protein and a vegetarian diet.

When not in a balanced state of health, the body of a B will either react like the O who's deprived of protein and become fatigued, or like the A, who produces excessive amounts of mucus. Type B individuals generally have a strong constitution and good autoimmune system. They can tolerate moderate amounts of dairy products, but if they eat or were fed excessive amounts of milk, cheese, and butter as children, they, like the A, will frequently suffer with catarrh (excessive mucus generally caused by an inflammation of the mucous membranes, particularly in the nose and throat). They may also be prone to respiratory diseases, food allergies, sinus problems, and asthma.

While I don't believe in drinking an excessive amount of coffee, one cup a day—preferably from organic coffee beans—and drunk black, will be fine for a B. Coffee turns increasingly acidic by adding milk and sugar to it, so if a B is in an imbalanced state of health, those few drops of milk in a cup of coffee can lead to colds, chronic coughs, and more serious respiratory problems.

And if a B lives in an environment that's heavily dependent on central heating or air-conditioning—both of which suck moisture from the air and dry the membranes lining the nasal passages, making them more irritable than normal—the mixture of dairy and dry passages will inflame the nasal passages and produce congestion. It's the same story for B's with skin ailments like eczema and psoriasis: mucus-forming foods and dry air will exacerbate their skin and worsen irritations.

Like the A, the B doesn't tolerate whole-wheat products well. Wheat substitutes like spelt, quinoa, and amaranth, and pastas made from rice would be preferable. Like the O, the B requires animal protein and can choose from many foods including turkey, lamb, salmon, and halibut. A Type B in a balanced state of health can also choose meals from a variety of vegetables and grains—the key is moderation.

Only about 7 percent of my patients are Type B's, but they're the easiest for me to identify of all the blood groups. Even before drawing a patient's blood, I can tell whether the person before me is a B. This blood type emerged from the East and is common among Semites and Asians, but I'm not referring to ethnicity when I say that this is an easily identifiable blood type. I'm talking about their disposition, character traits, and that certain indefinable something that gives Type B's their distinctive air.

The best way I can describe the B is someone who's highly practical yet who has one foot firmly planted in the spiritual world as well. These individuals seem to straddle the corporeal and transcendent worlds, melding them to bring a unique perspective to life.

Unlike A's, who tend to be more artsy or dreamlike in their spirituality, B's have a down-to-earth way about them. Part of this is their need for order. Whether it's their work space, home environment, or approach to problem solving, they thrive on organization and being methodical. This isn't to say that they suffer from a compulsive disorder. But disruptions can unsettle and upset them. Their ability to strategize and bring their world quickly under control is the hallmark of this blood type.

This characteristic serves B individuals well—it's what makes them born leaders, those who function best in positions of great responsibility. Type B's who don't hold positions of responsibility and leadership will live very frustrated lives. Because they tend to see solutions, not problems, they are dynamic innovators.

Exercise is less important for the B than for the O, although more important than it is for the A. Here, moderation is again an important word. B's tend to do well with brisk walking, swimming, hatha yoga, or light jogging. Whereas O's require an hour of aerobic exercise, B's should do no more than 30 minutes a day. After that, their bodies will start to feel fatigued.

Type B's fare well in competitive sports, such as basketball or tennis, but as the brain rules over brawn, they wouldn't find success as long-distance runners. But they perform exceptionally well in sports that require a creative and strategic mind. While they may not have the endurance of an O, the combination of physical strength and creativity can overcome that deficit and help them defeat an O.

Midpoint between O and A, B's who eat and exercise according to their blood type will enjoy a better-than-average life expectancy.

Type AB

The newest and rarest of the blood types, AB individuals constitute about 2 percent of the world population and possess the qualities of both A and B types. Anthropologists tell us that Type B's, the dominant type of people in the East, invaded the Roman Empire; intermarried with Type A's, who were the dominant type in Europe; and produced this last and newest of all blood types.

AB's inherited the tolerances of both A and B; and when in a balanced state of health, their immune systems tend to have an enhanced capacity to produce antibodies against infections. As a result, they're less prone to the allergic conditions and the autoimmune weaknesses typically seen in an A.

The best preventive diet is a mixture of the A and B diets. People who are Type AB do well on a diet geared toward vegetarianism, with the modest additions of some animal protein. Like Type A's, they don't tolerate dairy foods and are similarly subject to mucus production and respiratory conditions. Dairy products—cheese, milk, butter, and so forth—should be greatly reduced or entirely eliminated. Like the B, the AB can't tolerate whole wheat and should substitute it with products made from spelt, amaranth, quinoa, and rice flour.

Like Type A, AB's have a more active mind than body, although they tend to be slightly stronger constitutionally and more physically active. The perfect balance is 15 to 20 minutes of aerobic exercise at night to obtain cardiovascular benefits, and yoga in the morning to create the inner peace and calmness they require.

If Type B's are recognized for their unique sense of organization and A's for their spiritual and intellectual qualities, AB's possess qualities not frequently seen in any of the blood types. They can balance the creativity of the A and the grounded business sense of the B. Artistic people know the difficulty of staying practical while in the state of creation, and all corporate CEOs understand the internal struggle with their sensitive sides.

Those who are AB, a blood type that's still in infancy in terms of its evolution, seem to have this enormous talent of balancing the two worlds. *Balance* is a key word here. It's because of their sense of balance, not just in body but also in mind, that I believe AB individuals hold the fate of the human race in their blood. They have within them, not the apocalyptic notion and sad demise of the world, but the sense of peace and nonviolence that can help all of us move into an era of positive transformation.

I've often been accused of wearing rose-colored glasses, but as I view humanity through blood types and see the AB's as the next step in our evolution, I have great hope for the future, in spite of the threat of climate change, terrorism, and ongoing social and political unrest in the world.

≈ ≈ ≈

CHAPTER FOUR

Variations on a Theme: Sub–Blood Groups

Not long after I wrote *One Man's Food,* I went through a period in which I started to question my approach to individual diagnosis. Although I had established the idea of using the four blood groups as a methodology for diagnosing and treating patients—and had successfully healed many patients of chronic disorders—I began to wonder whether there were more than the four primary blood types. Patients have two parents, two sets of grandparents, four sets of great-grandparents and so on; and they don't all have the same blood type. Could there be slight variations because of the "mixing" of the different types?

For instance, would a patient with a parent whose blood type was O and another parent whose blood type was A have a dominant blood type, say the O, but with traits from the other A? In other words, could an O, who is meant to be active and energetic, but who has an A trait, prefer yoga? Could a Type B, who is highly organized and more business oriented, possess similar subtraits and be an artist who lives in a loft with paintings strewn about the studio?

If this were the case, then are blood groups really hybrids composed of more than one type instead of being monotypes?

Once I started on this line of thinking, I began to scrutinize patients in an even more critical way. I knew that my use of blood types—in conjunction with my diagnostic techniques of reading the iris and taking the six pulses—provided me with significant data with which to detect weaknesses in the body and then prescribe foods, herbs, vitamins, and assorted therapies to revitalize it. But if this were the case, if the blood types were really combinations of traits from different types, then I had to become more sensitive to the hybrids and prescribe even more in-depth menus to help heal and prevent diseases.

But how would I know this? When scientists have an intuitive feeling or a hunch that they may be on the verge of discovering something (or even discovering something new about their original finding), they might not know what they're looking for—only that they need to probe, investigate, and be open to variations or entirely new discoveries. So I followed up my initial hunch by developing a series of questions that might help me understand a person's individuality and particular needs better.

One of the first patients in whom I detected an anomaly was an internationally known photographer whose blood type was O. And yet, oddly, he presented very few O characteristics. He couldn't tolerate heavy exercise or dairy products. He was exceptionally sensitive and favored a vegetarian lifestyle. I reviewed his blood type several times, as this posed a direct challenge to my theory of individualization through the four blood groups. When I scrutinized his blood through magnification instead of just my naked eye, I noticed something I hadn't seen before.

Typically, when I type blood, I use two sera, the yellow B serum and a blue A serum. If the blood doesn't clot when it blends with either serum, the person has Type O blood. If the blood clots with the blue serum but not the yellow, the person has Type A blood. If it clots with the yellow but not the blue serum, the person is a Type B; and if it clots with both, the person has Type AB blood.

When I retested this patient's blood, it wasn't clotted in either serum, verifying that he was an O type. But then I noticed that the blood that had blended with the blue serum had fine clots around the outer edges, and I started to wonder if this wasn't the signature of another, less-dominant subtype group. Could an individual have more than one blood type—that is, a dominant type with traits of sub–blood groups? That concept certainly worked for this patient and his Type A qualities. When I re-created his menu, one that considered his A traits, he responded much better: the swelling in his joints and his painful arthritic condition started to abate.

I knew I had to go back to the drawing board and refine the blood-type concept and menus to include the possibility of the variations because of sub–blood group traits. Doing so would help me explain why some Type A's required rigorous sport activities beyond yoga, why some Type O's were hypersensitive and preferred quiet environments, and why some B's preferred a more solitary lifestyle.

I first became aware of the sub–blood groups in 1987 and have since incorporated them in diagnosis and menu planning for thousands of patients. There are six subtypes: Type Oa, Type Ob, Type Ao, Type Ab, Type Bo, and Type Ba. (The first letter, which is capitalized, indicates the primary blood type; and the lower-cased second letter represents the sub–blood group. To cite the earlier example of my patient: although his primary blood type was O, he exhibited dominant traits of Type A. I soon realized that a diet plan solely for Type O's wasn't working for him. Therefore, I included beneficial aspects for Type A's in his treatment, and I classified my patient as Type Oa.)

The combination of blood type and sub–blood type have helped me refine my analysis of my patients' particular needs when they're in the highest state of health or when recovering from an illness. I haven't found the sub–blood groups to be as standardized as the primary four blood types. If I can compare blood types to colors, I would say that O, A, B, and AB are like primary colors such as red, blue, yellow, and green.

The subgroups have different strengths or tones; and when blended with the primary colors, they produce different shades, such as when you mix a touch of yellow with red and get orange, or a blue to a green and get an aqua color. The sub–blood groups act to modify the primary shade, or blood group. And depending on the strength of the sub–blood group, it might produce different strengths and variations in the primary blood type. It's difficult to identify the variations in a person's blood type without thoroughly examining a blood sample under magnification. However, the following are a series of questions that I use in my diagnosis and which you can similarly put to use to further identify your primary blood type and the presence of a sub–blood type.

Type Oa

1. Were you subject to frequent colds and respiratory problems as a child? Do you suffer from these conditions now?

2. Do you currently have any allergies? Have you ever suffered from allergies?

3. Do you have asthma or suffer from sinusitis? Have you in the past?

4. Do you have a thyroid problem?

5. Does reading entice you more than physical exercise?

6. Are your hands and feet cold much of the time, even in hot weather?

7. Are you fatigued after exercising?

8. Are you allergic to dairy products?

9. Do you have problems with your gallbladder when you eat an excessive amount of meat?

10. Are you creative?

11. Do you have arthritis?

12. If you are a woman, do you have frequent vaginal discharge?

13. Does a sauna or hot bath fatigue you?

14. Are you sensitive to other people's problems?

If you answered *yes* to six or more of these questions and you're a Type O, then you're probably Type Oa. So if you read the previous chapter on blood types and thought that excessive exercise isn't right for you, you're correct. You are no marathoner. You should moderate your workouts, and if you're a runner, for instance, limit your distance to two to four miles per day. In addition, it would be wise to integrate yoga into your daily routine to help calm your nervous system.

You should also exclude dairy products from your diet, especially if you've developed any chronic respiratory conditions. You can eat some veal, lamb, and beef; but you should mostly eat fish. It's essential that you also read the section in this book about Type A, particularly the part about the A's mind. It will help broaden your understanding of your thought processes and your need to develop a meditation practice.

Type Ob

1. Are people drawn to you?

2. Do people often want to tell you about their troubles?

3. Do you enjoy working in the center of an organization, or do you own your own business?

4. Do you suffer from an allergy?

5. Could you somewhat tolerate being a vegetarian?

6. Would you rather counsel people with a problem than do rigorous exercise?

7. Do you have a broad range of unrelated interests?

8. Does disorder upset you?

9. Are you a strategic athlete as opposed to one who relies on pure brawn?

10. Do you have difficulty digesting tomatoes?

If you answered *yes* to four or more questions (or more than those for the Oa), you're probably Type Ob. You should reduce your dairy intake, but you can eat a wide variety of flesh foods including fish, some chicken, veal, lamb, and occasionally beef. Physical exercise is essential for you. You should also familiarize yourself with the section in this book on Type B blood.

Type Ao

1. Do you experience fatigue after three months of a vegetarian diet?

2. Does heavy physical exercise invigorate you?

3. Are you bothered by colds or chronic sinusitis?

4. Do you enjoy a sauna or hot bath?

5. Does physical exercise stimulate your mind?

6. Do you suffer from circulatory conditions?

7. Do you become nervous or stressed from overexercising?

8. Does exercise help you solve problems?

If you answered *yes* to questions 1, 2, 5, 6, and 8 and *no* to questions 3, 4, and 7, you're probably Type Ao. You will always require fish, chicken, lamb, and some veal in your diet; and if your lifestyle is highly physical, you'll probably need to consume flesh food daily. Your workout regimen should include about 20 minutes of yoga as well as 15 minutes of heavy exercise every day. Read the section on Type O to understand your physical needs.

Type Ab

1. Do dairy products upset your body?

2. Did you have frequent colds or respiratory problems as a child?

3. Do you enjoy running a business?

4. Do you enjoy group situations or activities?

5. Are you a magnetic person—that is, are people easily attracted to you?

6. Are you able to communicate ideas well?

7. Do you crave physical activities?

8. Do you like order in your life?

9. Do you motivate people?

10. Do people feel intimidated by you at times?

11. Do you struggle between always wanting to see the good in others versus needing to be cautious?

If you answered *yes* to more than six of these questions, you're probably Type Ab. These people exhibit Type A energy but can function well in a decision-making occupation. You may eat dairy products in very small amounts, fish and chicken sparingly (once a week), and lamb and buffalo once a month. You should be a vegetarian three or four days a week. Although you do require physical exercise, you need less than Type Ao.

Type Bo

1. Are you competitive in sports?

2. Do you like to strategize or conduct business while playing a sport?

3. Do you have a strong leaning toward flesh foods?

4. Do you enjoy debates?

5. Do you solve problems while exercising?

6. Would you rather take a vacation that included vigorous sporting activities than one that consisted of lying on the beach?

7. Do you own your own business, or do you have a key role in the business you are in?

If you answered *yes* to four or more questions, you're probably Type Bo. These are highly physical individuals who could run five to ten miles per day and who would excel in competitive sports. They are enthusiastic people who work well with others and enjoy participating in group activities and organizations. They're also the type who communicate better while exercising. So if you're a Type Bo who's carrying out a complex business negotiation, my advice is to do it on the golf course.

You should have access to a gym and engage in physical exercise before making important decisions. Dairy products can be enjoyed with minimal cutbacks, and flesh foods can be tolerated very well. However, you shouldn't eat chicken more than once a month.

Type Ba

1. Do you reach decisions when you're most relaxed?

2. Do quiet environments help you make decisions?

3. Do hyperactive people upset you?

4. Do you prefer yoga to running?

5. Do you gravitate toward being a vegetarian?

6. Do you prefer subdued colors around you, such as blues and greens?

7. Do you currently have allergies or sinus and mucous problems?

8. Does exercising for more than 35 minutes fatigue you?

If you answered *yes* to four or more questions, you're probably Type Ba. These individuals have all the qualities of Type B and considerable reservoirs of Type A's creativity. Respiratory problems —such as chronic colds, allergies, and sinusitis—are a lifelong challenge for these people; and they may also suffer from a variety of circulatory problems.

Dairy products need to be entirely removed from your diet, and whole-wheat products should be replaced by sprouted wheat and soy-based foods. Chicken should be eaten only one or two times a month, but fish is tolerated much more easily and can be eaten several times a week. Lamb and buffalo can be eaten in moderation. Exercise should include yoga or tai chi.

Once you know your blood type and determine your sub–blood type, you'll be able to zero in on your specific nutritional and exercise needs. This information will not only help you maintain good health and prevent a host of degenerative diseases, but if you're suffering from any of the conditions I describe in the next two chapters, this knowledge will help you overcome them and work your way back to an optimal state of well-being.

CHAPTER FIVE

Hypoglycemia— the Cause of Causes

Are you feeling as well as you should?

Do you wake up after eight hours of sleep feeling robust and energetic, clearheaded, and excited about the day? Or are you drowsy and irritable?

Are you struggling with something more serious than chronic colds or seasonal allergies? Have you developed pains in your joints or high cholesterol? Are you overweight, bouncing unsuccessfully from one diet plan to another?

Have you been diagnosed with adrenal fatigue? Fibromyalgia or chronic exhaustion? An autoimmune disease like rheumatoid arthritis?

Has your doctor told you that your hormonal levels are off? Is your menstrual cycle irregular? Do you have prolonged menstrual flows, or have you experienced difficulties getting pregnant?

Worse, have you discovered lumps in your breasts or somewhere else in your body?

Why do you think you've developed these or other such conditions?

Bad luck, you may say. Or it's in your genes and you believe you're preprogrammed to endure failing health. Perhaps it's owing to pollution and exposure to chemical contaminants, the goose liver you ate last Christmas, or possibly the eight eggs a week with bacon and home fries?

The only wrong answer in that list is the first one. Certainly, genetic disposition impacts health, as does living in a smoggy city or by an oil- or coal-refining plant. I think we all know at this point that high cholesterol and fatty foods are artery cloggers and can lead to heart disease. But luck? *Bzzzzzz . . . wrong answer.*

From my point of view, you are largely responsible for your current condition. If you have any kind of ailment, you, in part, created it. Yes, the cold; yes, the high cholesterol; yes, the arthritic pains; and yes, the cancer. And although it's true that many of these conditions are an outgrowth of your genetic makeup, did they necessarily have to come to life and manifest in your body?

Sure, that oil refinery down the road belching fumes and toxins will damage your lungs; in fact, environmental toxins are more prevalent in the air and water than ever before and are causative agents of disease. However, for the most part, that bag of groceries I talked about earlier (the one filled with foods that are completely inappropriate for you and your particular blood type and sub–blood group) is your main enemy. Trust me. I've been diagnosing and treating patients long enough and have seen too many people stumble blindly through their daily diet—the true cause of many physical, mental, and even emotional complaints.

Unnecessary Fatigue and Depression

Several years ago, a young man from New York came to see me complaining of being tired and depressed most of the time. The depression had limited his friendships, alienated him from his family, and greatly impeded his progress at his job in an advertising firm. This isn't surprising—a person with a low energy level and melancholy disposition is hardly going to be the life of a party, an enthusiastic colleague at the workplace, or one who's able to manage the complex relationships in a family.

I diagnosed him as having low blood sugar and greatly reduced his intake of high-density carbohydrates such as potatoes, pastas, and bakery goods. As he was an O, I oriented him more to a high-protein diet. It didn't take long in his particular case to normalize his blood-sugar levels. Several months of the diet achieved that. He saw a remarkable turnaround in his energy level and his state of mind, followed by a new attitude in his communication at work and with his family.

Here is where I'll use the word that I previously said didn't apply to health: he was a *lucky* one. Lucky only in that he caught his condition early before it did the kind of damage that low blood sugar, otherwise known as hypoglycemia, can do to a person's body. Approximately 85 to 90 percent of my patients are hypoglycemic, including those who also suffer from obesity, diabetes, hormonal imbalances, infertility, ADD, alcoholism, coronary disease, and cancer.

Low blood sugar is not only the most common cause of disease in the majority of my patients, but also the shadow or underlying cause of most degenerative diseases. Uncontrollable levels of sugar in the body gradually wear down the pancreas, which is constantly forced to produce insulin to neutralize and balance these levels. For most people, the disposition to hypoglycemia was probably carried over genetically from the grandparents, who either had a significantly weakened pancreas or diabetes. Hypoglycemia is a precursor to diabetes, and if not treated will eventually lead to that disease.

A weakened pancreas also stresses the adrenal glands, which impacts its production of cortisol. Once the adrenal glands are debilitated and no longer produce adequate cortisol, it can lead to the sorry story of biochemical imbalance that can result in a broad range of diseases, including arthritis, autoimmune deficiency, and the hormonal deficiencies that disrupt a woman's menstrual cycle and prevent conception.

Hypoglycemia—an Octopus with Many Arms

Hypoglycemia is the scourge of our time, as its tentacles reach out to many other parts of the body.

I'm not the first to address this—in fact, the damaging effects of low blood sugar have been known for decades. Where I differ is in the treatment of hypoglycemia and its accompanying diseases and, of course, in its prevention.

For most people, the condition probably started in childhood—these individuals consumed processed foods, those laced with preservatives and an exaggerated amount of complex carbohydrates, and foods loaded with sugar (or, more recently, with sweetening substitutes like fruit juices, sugarcane extract, and high-fructose corn syrup). These foods not only failed to nourish, but started these children down the path to obesity. Moreover, they compromised the biochemical relationships among enzymes, hormones, and normal cellular life.

Let me be very clear about this: nourishment from early childhood onward determines the quality of health a person will experience as a toddler, adolescent, adult, and senior. Our bodies are made up of trillions of cells, and each cell has a differentiated job—it knows what it must do in the body. A kidney cell, for example, doesn't err and suddenly start acting like a liver cell. Our DNA has determined what our cells will do. RNA, another component of a cell, is the taskmaster that carries out the DNA's orders. RNA makes sure that each new cell is an exact replica of the cell it replaces, but in order for the cells to replicate perfectly, they require nourishment.

And this is where things begin to go awry for most people, especially those who have hypoglycemia, who have blindly added sugar or honey to their foods and mistakenly believed that the energizing jolt from a sweetened food or a sandwich made of thick bread with fries on the side—or even a fruit smoothie or carrot juice—would give them a boost and get them through long hours at work. It's even worse for individuals who turn to shots of whiskey or a half-dozen beers after work to relieve stress or help them get through a crisis.

You can take it to the bank that all people who have relied on a long-term diet of carbohydrates and sugars feel fatigued when they wake up, are increasingly lackluster by late morning, and need a nap generally right after lunch or by midafternoon. This is because they have weakened themselves at the cellular level, and weakened cells create weakened organs (kidneys, adrenal glands, pancreas, liver, and so on) and a weakened immune system.

What I've found exciting—no, enthralling—and what has kept me passionately involved in healing, is the body's remarkable resilience: its ability, in many cases, to regenerate and recover its strength and vitality. Just as the wrong foods can produce weak cells that are susceptible to degenerative diseases, proper nourishment can reverse the process and produce strengthened cells that nourish and keep the body healthy. Even cells with genetic dispositions to diseases such as arthritis or heart disease can be revitalized.

It takes time and real work to repair the damage that has occurred in your cells, and even more work to repair the damage caused by previous generations and transmitted to you through DNA. Whether you're new to my work or are a practitioner who has tried to apply my principles of individual diagnosis and treatment, it's essential that the patient who has hypoglycemia—or any condition—is respected as an individual with unique bodily needs. This is where I differ in the treatment of hypoglycemia, diabetes, coronary disease, obesity, and other conditions tangled in its web.

Are You Hypoglycemic?

If you or your children have not been identified as having hypoglycemia—it's often overlooked by medical doctors—I would recommend that you review the classic symptoms right now. If you experience ongoing fatigue, sugar cravings, depression, irritability, and dips in energy levels at around 11 A.M. or between 2 and 3 P.M.; and if you feel the need for a Coke or coffee, a candy bar, or even a protein bar by midafternoon to pick you up, odds are you're suffering from hypoglycemia.

There are limits to what a reader can derive from a book, but if any of these symptoms are prevalent, you should follow the hypoglycemia-treatment diet at the end of this chapter.

If you are a Type O, it will take two to two-and-a-half years to cure hypoglycemia. It takes up to three years for a Type A, and two-and-a-half to three years to correct the condition in a Type B. But by following my program, you can correct this condition so that if you're of childbearing age, you won't pass it along to your children and will lessen the chance of them developing hypoglycemia or diabetes; if you're beyond childbearing age, you can go into your senior years with renewed health and vitality, avoiding many of the common degenerative diseases of advancing years.

(*Please note:* All diets should always be adhered to under the guidance of a qualified medical doctor or other type of health-care practitioner with knowledge and ample experience in applying the D'Adamo blood type and sub–blood type method.)

If you don't experience any of the symptoms of hypoglycemia, then follow the diet for your blood and sub–blood groups laid out in the diet sheets and daily menus (which are located in Chapters 7 and 8). They can help prevent the condition from ever occurring. Remember, the blood type and sub–blood type diets are manuals that direct you to the foods your individual body requires to maximize your health.

My diagnosis for hypoglycemia—and all disease—begins by employing a combination of iridology, pulse diagnosis, and blood typing, which includes an analysis of Rh factors and other blood indicators (A1's and H1's). The diagnosis is actually an interplay between these three methods. By taking the pulses first, I get a general idea of a person's current weaknesses. Blood typing and sub–blood typing allow me to focus my attention on a person's specific makeup and what their condition should be if they are in a perfect state of health.

An examination of the iris, which outwardly reflects the inner weaknesses of the body, helps validate the other two techniques. Using the three approaches helps me understand the *cause* of the symptoms—not just the symptoms—and what specific menu, exercise plan, supplements, and additional therapies are needed to reverse the causes.

Even without these diagnostic techniques, hypoglycemia is so prevalent that I assume the majority of my patients between the ages of 3 and 50 have developed some form of sugar intolerance and are in a state of chronic fatigue. I see it right away in their faces—they often look spent and worn-out, as if they haven't had a really good night's sleep in years. Even the patients who have some spunk are masking an artificially induced energy or an irritability or depression that I detect when I look more deeply.

I don't have to ask what their current diet is, but when I do, it's almost always the same for all of my patients: two-thirds of the person's diet consists of sugar and starch in the form of potatoes, bread, pasta, rice, and some fruits and vegetables. Most Americans' palates have become so accustomed to carbohydrates—whether it's the cereal, toast, or croissant for breakfast; the roll that comes on the side of a mixed-green salad; the drizzle of chocolate syrup on an ice-cream sundae; the squirt of maple syrup on a stack of buttermilk pancakes; the touch of honey in a cup of chamomile tea; or that pint of beer or glass of red wine after work—that they can't pass a day without them.

Taken in moderation, any of the above items might not have a damaging effect on the body. But most people in the U.S. don't feel satisfied after meals unless they finish them off with something sweet or loaded with carbs.

I'll give you the bad news and tough love up front so you know what you're getting yourself into should you try to reverse your hypoglycemia: the five to eight weeks it will take to kick your addiction to sugar will be about as difficult a time as you've ever experienced in your life. But unless you can rein in your consumption of sugars and carbohydrates, the sugar intolerance will continue and further compromise your body beyond the damage to your adrenal glands and pancreas, which have taken the hardest hits from this disease. You will continue down the road of declining health.

The choice is yours.

Recommendations for Treating Hypoglycemia

1. Entirely eliminate all sources of sugar sweeteners: white or brown sugar, honey, molasses, maple syrup, and all artificial sweeteners.

2. Eliminate soft drinks and all sources of alcohol—this means beer, wines, hard liquor such as brandy and whiskey, and all mixed drinks like mojitos, daiquiris, and martinis.

3. Severely reduce your daily intake of bread, rice, or pasta. Don't eat more than one-half to one slice of bread per day (and that includes whole-wheat bread).

4. Reduce or eliminate vegetables with a high sugar content such as carrots, potatoes, beetroot, and onions.

5. Reduce or eliminate fruits with a high sugar content such as apples, pineapples, cherries, and bananas.

Daily Diets

There are 21 primary meals in a week, and all of them should contain portions of protein. Type O's would lean toward the heavier animal proteins such as buffalo, beef, lamb, and occasionally fish. Type A's and AB's would lean toward the lighter protein, such as fish, turkey, and occasionally lamb or chicken. (Note that Type A individuals can't tolerate a vegetarian diet until their sugar intolerance is cured.) Type B's can integrate both heavy and light protein at their meals. All blood types must supplement their main meals with high-protein snacks.

Here's what a daily menu should look like (all blood types):

Upon rising, squeeze half a lemon into an 8-ounce glass of tepid water and drink. Types O and B should then exercise for 20 minutes. Types A and AB should practice yoga. Follow your workout with an energy drink. A high-protein drink for O's and B's should consist of:

- 1 Tbsp. hydrolyzed whey powder

- 2 Tbsp. lecithin granules

- 1 tsp. stractan, an herb from the larch tree (optional)

- 1 tsp. yeast

- 4 to 5 oz. water or rice milk; substitute with grapefruit juice once a week

Types A and AB should use the same formula, but eliminate the yeast and substitute soy for whey powder. Breakfast should follow. Types O and B can eat:

- ½ grapefruit
- A protein drink or one egg
- Herbal tea

Types A and AB can also have some kind of spelt, quinoa, or puffed rice with soy milk. Two or three days a week, they may substitute an egg or the protein drink for the cereal.

At about 11 A.M., eat a stalk of celery or a rice cake smeared with almond butter. Or eat a handful of almonds or sunflower seeds.

Lunch should consist of a salad of six or seven vegetables as well as tofu, fish, turkey, beef, lamb (occasionally), or buffalo, depending on your blood type. Finish with herbal tea.

At 2 P.M., eat a snack of almonds and sunflower seeds, or have another celery stalk or rice cake with almond butter or tofu.

At 6 P.M., eat a meal of meat, fish, turkey, or chicken and at least three to five vegetables.

Between 9 and 10 P.M., have another protein shake because it's vital to maintain a relatively normal blood-sugar level. Drinking a shake at this point will prevent your level from lowering throughout the night and help reduce the early-morning fatigue and irritability that are so common to hypoglycemia.

It's also essential to avoid eating any foods with high carbohydrate contents for dinner, such as pasta or rice. They will trigger a fluctuation in your blood-sugar level while you sleep and negatively affect your mood and energy when you wake up.

Vitamins

Vitamins should be taken by all blood types. Note that the daily vitamin regimen for hypoglycemia should be broad and comprehensive and include B complex, niacin, B_6, zinc, chromium, selenium, iron, vitamin C, and pancreatic tablets. A vitamin guide for prevention and healing appears later in the book (in Chapter 12) and is organized by blood type and sub–blood type. It can be used as a full-reference guide for hypoglycemia.

Words of Advice and Encouragement

Be very patient. It took you years to create the hypoglycemia, and depending upon your current condition and any other underlying conditions that may exist, you'll need to follow a strict diet before you begin to experience a resurgence of energy. But it *can* be done. Thousands of my patients have followed my recommendations and have regained their full health and vitality. If you can't adhere to the program 100 percent (I know that people find convenient excuses and go off their diets from time to time), you'll recover your vitality proportionate to your effort. In other words, if you follow the diet 85 percent of the time, that's how much health you can expect to restore.

A Bit More Advice

During your first three or four weeks, you may experience headaches, stomachaches, or fatigue. Don't be concerned. Your body has been addicted to foods you've eaten for many years and is rebelling against the new diet. You're getting rid of old habits, but old habits die hard.

CHAPTER SIX

Treating Hypoglycemia-related Diseases

As I said in the previous chapter—and let me reemphasize this—*hypoglycemia is highly treatable.* If you have Type O blood, it can take two to two-and-a-half years to cure it; for Type A, it can take up to three years to regain full health; and Type B falls somewhere in between the O and A time frames. But once cured, once no longer enslaved by your body's craving for sugar and carbohydrates, you'll be able to enjoy foods such as pasta, bread, and rice; and even drink red wine, all according to your blood type.

Be warned: when you first go on the program, the initial weeks will be difficult, as you have to refrain from eating what you love because those particular foods have created your current condition. Your body wants you to eat those foods; and as you adopt a new diet, you may experience stomachaches, headaches, or fatigue.

But there is a payoff: In time, you'll experience a resurgence of physical energy and mental clarity. Moreover, you will have prevented the further weakening of your body's organs, systems, and defenses, which inevitably opens the door to an onslaught of any number of degenerative diseases.

Once fully cured, you ensure your own robust health into your senior years.

But what happens if you don't cure hypoglycemia? What can you expect?

Let me show what occurs when sugar-filled products, chocolate shops, ice-cream parlors, soda machines, and fast-food joints come to town.

In the mid-1990s, researchers started to analyze and praise the Mediterranean diet, which has been the staple diet in countries that bordered the Mediterranean for centuries. Because people in this region had lower rates of serious diseases than many Americans, and on average lived longer, their dietary habits were of special interest.

The Mediterranean diet is low in saturated fats and high in nutrients derived from vegetables; and is also heavy on fruit, unrefined grains, olive oil, and wine, which is consumed in moderation on a daily basis. Fish, eggs, and chicken are a small part of the diet, eaten once or twice a week. The key, too, is that processed foods (refined sugar and flour, butter, and other fats) are rarely consumed.

However, in the past decade, health officials, including those from the Food and Agriculture Organization of the United Nations, have grown alarmed by a new phenomenon in the Mediterranean region: people are getting sick—very sick—in ways they never have. Interestingly, the diseases aren't manifesting in the adult population, those who have been adhering to the Mediterranean diet. Rather, it's the children who are suddenly falling prey to a sequence of degenerative diseases more commonly associated with middle age.

As reported in *The New York Times* in September 2008, childhood ailments are now being overshadowed by diabetes, high cholesterol, high blood pressure, kidney stones, and the scourge of the American diet: obesity. Two-thirds of all children in Greece are now overweight and are living shorter lives in comparison to their parents, who still adhere to the Mediterranean diet!

Why? Because over the last ten years, convenience stores and supermarkets started to appear in even the smallest villages of southern European countries, bringing with them seemingly innocuous processed foods: cereals with high sugar content, frozen pizza, ice cream, candy, and sodas containing high-fructose corn syrup. The kind of food that bloats and poisons many Americans.

In less than a generation, Mediterranean children, who have adopted an American-style diet, are suffering extreme health-related problems—*not* their parents.

The Mediterranean diet has now become the "Mediterranean Nightmare"; and is a new, living, and dramatic model of the severe impact of excessive sugar and carbohydrates on a society. Could all of this have been prevented?

I can offer up many case histories—sad case histories—of people I've treated or advised regarding their nutritional habits and the impact of low blood sugar on their health. Naysayers may raise an eyebrow or two; even those who are disposed to following the D'Adamo diet are sometimes skeptical about my claims and the impact of hypoglycemia.

I would encourage those who are skeptical or who say they've heard all this before to put aside their doubts and take to heart this new paradigm of disease spreading across the Mediterranean. Then they should also think about their own eating habits (especially when reaching for the double scoop of ice cream or second helping of linguine), and consider the impact these foods will have on their health. Tragically, many of these Greek children have gone the route of hypoglycemia and have no idea that they're facing a life of serious, chronic diseases.

This, I think, answers the question of what happens and what one can expect if hypoglycemia is not cured.

I've touched on a physiological domino effect—that is, the sequence of events that can happen in the body once hypoglycemia develops—in previous chapters, but I'll repeat the implications and impact of hypoglycemia before I offer suggestions for preventing and/or treating some of the offshoot diseases that can result.

For one thing, hypoglycemia is a precursor to diabetes (I'm referring to type 2 diabetes, not juvenile diabetes, which isn't a food-associated disease); and untreated hypoglycemia will invariably lead to diabetes, which is the extreme end point of this condition.

You may consider yourself hypoglycemic if your blood sugar is lower than 80 on a glucometer. As I said, when hypoglycemia goes untreated, the stress to the pancreas will ultimately weaken it and produce insulin deficiency, causing diabetes.

If you've been diagnosed with diabetes, you should work with a physician or qualified health practitioner and immediately follow the hypoglycemia diet (according to your blood and sub–blood types), as laid out in the previous chapter. The appropriate diet and exercise routine for your blood type can manage this condition and reduce the need for insulin (the blood-type diet is especially effective if you've had diabetes for less than ten years). But the impact of hypoglycemia goes beyond diabetes, and again, it's only the starting point for other degenerative diseases.

If the impact of your hypoglycemia has caused adrenal fatigue, in addition to debilitating the pancreas, then your level of cortisol, the body's natural corticosteroid, will be diminished. Reduced cortisol will first cause aches and pains in the joints and, as the condition progresses, eventually result in the corrosion of tissue in the joints and harrowing, disfiguring rheumatoid arthritis.

As we saw in the Mediterranean region, obesity is another direct result of hypoglycemia. Weight-reduction diets, as far as I'm concerned, do not work. People starve themselves to lose pounds, then go off the diet and put the weight right back on. The reason they go off their diets and regain the weight nine out of ten times is because of their addiction: the body's craving for sugar and carbohydrates.

Obesity and alcoholism, which I'll address momentarily, have the same root cause. Some people may be genetically disposed to weight gain. But those who shovel in cakes, cookies, ice cream, potato chips, pasta (and more pasta), and sugary fruit juices and soft drinks will eventually become so addicted to the sugar content that, in most cases, they put on excessive weight, while also polluting their bodies with a range of toxic substances.

As the pounds are added, every organ is strained: Waste products are cemented to the colon and within the tissues of the kidneys and liver, diminishing their capacity to clear the bloodstream and thereby poisoning the entire body. The heart and circulatory system labor to pump blood to all organs, systems, and body extremities, as fats and cholesterol glue themselves to arteries. Normal cells start feeding off accumulated toxic waste and foods that are devoid of nutritional value, endangering the integrity of these cells and setting the stage for them to become cancerous. Finally, of course, the pancreas and adrenal glands eventually run out of steam as they seek to regulate the body's blood sugar.

An obese body is tantamount to a small compact car lugging a huge Mack truck filled with tons of cargo—and it inevitably breaks down.

The alcoholic's body is faced with similar stress. Years ago I attended Alcoholics Anonymous (AA) meetings to study the diet of alcoholics. To their credit, the people I met at those meetings had suppressed their addiction to liquor. They met on a regular basis to lend support and help keep themselves alcohol free. But I noticed that at the end of each meeting, the group gathered around a coffee table to snack on sugary pastries and drink coffee, Coca-Cola, or other soft drinks. What they didn't realize was that their bodies couldn't differentiate between having a couple of stiff drinks or a Coke, in terms of the addictive qualities.

Of course, soft drinks don't take the edge off in the way that alcohol does; in fact, it does just the opposite. Soda produces a rush of sugar into the bloodstream, exciting the body with a false sense of energy. The addiction had never really changed.

Yes, many people may have a psychological dependence on alcohol, but the truth of the matter is that these individuals were feeding their bodies' craving for sugar.

Treating hypoglycemia is not only a treatment for alcoholism, it's also a preventive measure for the disease. People who are hypoglycemic are at a greater risk of developing an alcohol dependency because of their chronic need for a sugar fix. Many of my patients who were alcoholics not only ended their addiction to both sugar and alcohol, but went on to become social drinkers—including that glass of heart-friendly red wine for dinner.

But the impact of hypoglycemia is much greater than the havoc it creates in blood-sugar levels. As previously noted, it can weaken a woman's hormonal system, resulting in irregular menstruation cycles and difficulty conceiving; it can lead to ADD, depression, and other psychological conditions; and it's frequently at the root of coronary, liver, and urinary diseases. Finally, this condition can be so disturbing to the normal cell that it produces abnormal ones that reproduce abnormally, which is the physiological description of what occurs when you have the disease called cancer.

The following are additional measures you can take to treat the possible effects of hypoglycemia. All of these should be referred to in conjunction with the hypoglycemia menus for your blood type in the previous chapter, and under the guidance of a physician.

Diabetes (Type 2)

According to the American Diabetes Association, 23.6 million people in the United States, or 8 percent of the population, have diabetes. The rate of new cases rose by 14 percent between 2005 and 2007 alone, fueled by growing obesity and sedentary lifestyles. Diabetes experts say the findings show that there's no end in sight to this epidemic.

Controlling sugar and insulin levels is key to treating type 2 diabetes. All sugars and starches have to be kept to a minimum—people of all blood types should strictly adhere to the hypoglycemic diet for their blood type.

Insulin levels must be checked two to three times a day. The more insulin the person takes per day through medicine, the less insulin the body will produce. And that's the hook. An individual can become medically dependent on insulin, which will in turn reduce the functionality of the pancreas and inhibit its production of natural insulin.

Vitamins and herbal extracts can play an important part in the treatment of diabetes. I believe that vitamins should be regarded as a drug. They're recommended by physicians and health practitioners as generic supplements for all people, and although they can provide a quantity of nutrients the body may require, they may also be consumed in quantities that are inappropriate. In other words, not all people should take the same amount of multivitamins.

Follow the recommendations based on your blood type and sub–blood type (guidelines are located in Chapter 12), in addition to important vitamins listed here:

- *Multivitamins.* Type O's should take a high-stress formula, Type A's should take a low-stress formula, and Type B's can take a medium-strength formula.

- B_{12}. Type A's require a higher dose, and Types O and B require a lower amount.

- B_6. This vitamin is very important for circulation. Diabetics frequently develop circulatory problems.

- *Pancreas and adrenal extracts.* These extracts are important to revitalize both the pancreas and adrenal glands.

- *Calcium.* Type A's must take this in conjunction with hydrochloric-acid tablets to help assimilate the calcium.

- *Vanadium.* This vitamin helps the pancreas produce insulin.

The following therapies are also important in treating diabetes:

- German footbaths help improve circulation and may be available at European-style natural-healing clinics or spas. Commercially sold footbaths don't contain the same herbal combination nor do they effectively stimulate circulation.

- If a person has poor elimination, colonic irrigation can improve the functioning of the colon.

- Hyperbaric-chamber treatment pumps oxygen into the body, which helps bring more oxygen to the blood. This in turn increases oxygen to the cells, which helps release toxicity.

- Acupuncture is an effective way of improving circulation.

Obesity

The first question people have to ask themselves is: *Why am I obese?* Yes, there can be a genetic component involved, but in 95 percent of all my patients who struggle with excessive weight gain or obesity, the problem isn't genetics but hypoglycemia. Excessive weight or obesity is a symptom, not a cause, and almost always indicates an addiction to sugar and carbohydrates.

It is absolutely imperative—and I can't stress this enough— for those who struggle with excess weight to strictly adhere to the nutritional needs of their individual blood type and follow the specific hypoglycemic diet to a tee. I've treated thousands of patients after they tried Weight Watchers, Jenny Craig, or some other weight-reduction diet; and their single greatest complaint was that after all the many months of dieting, they eventually gained the weight back.

Follow the hypoglycemic menu for your blood type, increasing protein and drastically cutting all sources of carbohydrates and sugars. You must eat protein three times a day. Between meals, eat a small amount of almond butter on celery stalks or a handful of walnuts, sunflower seeds, or almonds. It's imperative to keep your protein level up and constant throughout the day. (Type A's can mix tofu and almond butter on celery sticks as a snack between meals.) Drink protein shakes in the morning based on your blood group (follow the recipe in the previous chapter).

Have another protein drink at 2 P.M. and before going to sleep at around 10 P.M. I also recommend that patients eat half a teaspoon of almond butter on celery before going to bed to maintain balanced sugar levels throughout the night. If you don't maintain your sugar level, you'll wake up feeling tired and possibly in a bad mood. And in the morning, the vicious hypoglycemic syndrome will be perpetuated as you try to satisfy the need for sugar with a doughnut, toast, or even a large portion of fruit or orange juice— all things with high-sugar or carbohydrate contents.

In addition, take B complex according to your blood type. Add vitamins C and E and lecithin, calcium, magnesium, and zinc. Adrenal and pancreas extracts are vital during this period to rebuild and support both glands.

Gymnema is an ayurvedic herb that can help with appetite management. Other therapies include colonics (to rid the body of stored-up putrefied waste), acupuncture, and a Firard sauna with oxygen. (A Firard machine generates infrared light waves that promote deep, penetrating heat, which unlike conventional infrared waves, aren't blocked at the body's surface. The Firard machine is often used to stimulate acupuncture needles in the treatment of lower back pain or to increase "yang" energy in the body.)

Of course, exercising (according to your blood type) in the morning will invigorate and stimulate your body and mind. In addition, it's essential to stay on the diet even as you start to lose weight. Yes, you will shed pounds on this diet, but that doesn't mean you've cured your hypoglycemia. Know that when you cure your hypoglycemia, you will cure your obesity. At that time, you'll be able to comfortably expand your diet without putting the weight back on.

One helpful hint: Look in the mirror and ask yourself if you want to remain overweight. The key is to love yourself more. You need to capture a positive image of yourself and reinforce this on a regular basis. You'll never attain your goal by idly wishing and hoping for a more normal body weight. You've abused yourself, but now is the time to love yourself and develop a more positive self-image.

Arthritis

Many forms of arthritis are the result of excessive sugar and/or carbs in the body, as well as stress. As the pancreas is stressed and weakened due to hypoglycemia, the adrenal glands are called into play to support the pancreas and forestall diabetes. Unfortunately, they eventually become exhausted and, as I explained, deplete the body's natural cortisol, which leads to arthritic conditions or fibro-myalgia.

As with all sugar-associated conditions, people suffering from the aches and pains and debilitating effects of arthritis must monitor their consumption of sugar and carbohydrates. In addition, they should take the following supplements according to their blood types:

- *Vitamins A and D* (I've found that a high dose of vitamin A without high doses of vitamin D can cause aches and pains. Vitamin A 10,000 IU should be balanced with 800–1,200 mg vitamin D, depending upon your blood type.)

- *Cod-liver oil*

- *Boswellia herb* (ayurvedic)

- *Glucosamine sulfate*

- *B complex* (according to your blood group)

- *Calcium with vitamin K*

Type A's must take hydrochloric-acid tablets with calcium. Colonics will help wash out wastes and uric acid stored in the lower colon, which, if not eliminated, eventually make their way into muscles and joints, causing arthritic conditions.

I also recommend acupuncture and chiropractic treatments for pain management and constitutional-hydrotherapy treatments, particularly for Type O's, to help eliminate toxins from the body.

Heart-Related Conditions

In order to maintain a healthy heart, a total shift in values in relation to food, work, stress, and physical exercise is required. High cholesterol (and its subsequent effects on coronary arteries), diabetes, obesity, and heart- and kidney-related conditions often develop together and are interrelated. Medical responses to coronary conditions, such as stents to expand and open clogged arteries and bypass-valve operations, are temporary fixes for the major problem: years of dietary abuse. Add stress, lack of exercise, and smoking, and you have the basic causes of most heart conditions.

Many heart-related conditions can be managed to a degree, but a person really has to decide how much health he or she wants to try to recover. The heart-related diet can be even more drastic than a hypoglycemic diet. All sugars and carbohydrates have to be greatly reduced, as do cheeses, dairy products, butter, fats, and protein consumption. Type A's will need to become exclusively vegetarians; Type O's will have to modify their normal intake of animal proteins, eating lean meats such as turkey, fish, and buffalo; and Type B's can eat turkey, fish, and some lamb with no fat.

Let me make it perfectly clear that I am absolutely against the use of cholesterol-reducing drugs. Cholesterol levels can be brought down through careful dietary changes and an exercise program. (Exercise programs according to your blood type are an essential part of a cholesterol-reducing diet and should be eased into very gradually.) Cholesterol-lowering drugs, however, come with a huge price to the liver and are really the lazy person's approach: drugs like statins allow people to continue gorging on food. But don't fool yourself. All medicines come with side effects. Just listen to a television ad for a cholesterol-reducing drug like Crestor, and you'll hear the long list of deleterious side effects.

Vitamins should include B complex, B_6, B_{12}, and especially E, which thins the blood. Lecithin helps clean the arteries; and Choleast, which is made from red yeast rice, also helps rid the body of cholesterol. Magnesium, zinc, CoQ10, neocarditone, and hawthorn berry are also important supplements to take at this time.

Chelation therapy can help reduce plaque from the arteries, and EPA 3 and 6 and cod-liver oil are vital to restoring flexibility to the arteries and reducing plaque.

High Blood Pressure

If you have high blood pressure, follow the same kind of diet for cholesterol according to your blood type, reducing heavy meats such as beef and pork, as well as dairy products. Salt should also be eliminated, along with foods high in sodium, such as celery or olives. Fluid intake must be increased to at least eight glasses of water a day. Eating garlic is also useful, as it naturally lowers blood pressure.

A wide range of therapies can be employed to cleanse the body, improve circulation, and reduce high blood pressure. Nattoki-nase, an enzyme created when soy is fermented, prevents platelet aggregation in the arteries and eases blood pressure. Colonics, footbaths, chiropractic or osteopathy, acupuncture, and multistep oxygen therapy can all be beneficial for this condition.

Vitamin C strengthens the walls of the arteries, and rutin tablets can also revitalize them. *Rauwolfia serpentina,* an herb long used in Indian ayurvedic medicine, can help reduce blood pressure; garlic and potassium intake, as well as drinking a lot of water, are also ways to get this condition under control.

Taking stock of your stress level is essential in treating high blood pressure. You may need to make lifestyle adjustments and adopt a more relaxing way of life. Exercise is helpful in reducing stress and improving this condition, but make no mistake about it: high blood pressure is a dangerous condition, and any changes you implement—whether they are dietary or in terms of physical exercise—must be supervised by a qualified physician.

Low Blood Pressure

Apart from the dietary changes previously mentioned, people with low blood pressure should take an array of vitamins including B complex, B_6, C, E, and A; along with B_{12}, folic acid, iron, and dessicated liver. Type A's should not take high-stress B vitamins and should stay within the recommended levels for vitamin C intake. In addition, niacin can be beneficial for this condition because it acts as a vasodilator (flushing of the face is frequently a normal response to niacin).

As low blood pressure is often caused by thyroid problems, everyone should have their thyroid gland checked. You may have an underactive thyroid gland and require some mild medication.

Cancer

Not all cancers are directly related to dietary abuse. Cancerous conditions can develop for a number of reasons, including stress, excessive exposure to sunlight, and the intake of harsh preservatives and chemicals. But cancer is largely a food-associated disease, although not every case is related to hypoglycemia and stress.

Poor nutritional habits, especially eating outside of the diet for your blood type, have two effects: they weaken the body by supplying inadequate nutrition, thereby weakening the immune system; and they increase toxicity levels. A body that has a high level of toxicity autointoxifies—in other words, cellular life becomes polluted by feeding off of toxins in the bloodstream. And that is how normal cells eventually become abnormal cells that reproduce at an abnormal rate, which is the definition of cancer.

Cancer is not caused by a germ, bacteria, or virus. It is an autoimmune disease produced by years of stress and nutritional abuse. And yes, there are specific foods that seem to stop the production of cancerous cells, like broccoli or cauliflower, but many green vegetables that aren't genetically modified or sprayed with pesticides are beneficial in stopping cancerous growths. Following a diet according to your blood type is truly the key to preventing this dreadful disease.

If hypoglycemia is detected, all blood types should adhere to the appropriate hypoglycemic diet for their type of blood. If you are not hypoglycemic, follow the normal diet for your blood type. Either way, you must include B complex, B_{12}, B_6, and vitamins A, D, and E as the core of your supplement program. If you are in fact hypoglycemic, you will need to take pancreatic enzymes at least five times a day to strengthen your pancreas.

The goal in treating cancer is to shrink the growths and stop the spread of abnormal cells. Diet alone will not achieve this, however. It is mandatory to detox and cleanse the body. Therapies that reduce the toxicity in the body include colonics, footbaths, and hyperbaric chamber. As cancer cells cannot live in the presence of oxygen or intense heat, I also employ the Firard sauna with oxygen and multistep oxygen therapy. (These are the standard therapies used at the D'Adamo Institute, although they may not all be available at many health clinics.) Intravenous feedings of high dosages of vitamin C with homeopathic mistletoe is an effective remedy for treating cancer in conjunction with agaricus and maitake mushrooms and pectins. If cancerous cells have spread to the liver, treatments can include liver tinctures, cod-liver oil, vitamin D, vitamin B_{12}, CoQ10, lots of pancreatic enzymes, and agaricus mushroom. It is vital to note that these supplements and vitamins must only be taken in consultation with a qualified physician.

Depression and Anxiety

If the bloodstream is an unsettled sea, the body and mind will feel as if they're a ship being tossed about by wave after crashing wave. The physiological and psychological implications of blood surging with sugar and excessive carbohydrates cannot be underestimated: if you are suffering from depression or any form of anxiety, you can be sure that your blood-sugar levels are at the root of the cause. Eliminating all sources of sugar and carbohydrates will calm your inner waters, and your mood swings and states of mind will level off almost immediately.

Along with an exercise program appropriate for your blood type, B complex, pantothenic acid, and vitamins B_6 and B_{12} are the core components for getting this condition under control. Herbs such as *Rhodiola rosea* can relax the adrenal glands, which in turn will decrease the body's stress and fatigue; and Saint-John's-wort or Passiflora, chamomile, skullcap, or valerian are also recommended. Acupuncture and German footbaths can also help calm and soothe the body.

If you're suffering from any kind of depression or anxiety, you should seek counseling immediately.

CHAPTER SEVEN

Menus for Blood Types and Sub– Blood Types

It's written in Jewish Law that "one should not eat according to the taste buds. Instead the foods to be eaten should be chosen wisely with an understanding of which foods will give strength to the entire body."

I've rarely met people who have a real intuitive sense of the foods they require. Most eat to satisfy their taste buds or to partake of the very latest and most highly advertised nouvelle cuisine.

This chapter contains seven-day starter menus for each blood type. I've prepared them to help you choose the appropriate foods for you, and to also help you ease into the program. I know that making changes can be demanding and, at times, confusing. But you will have an easier time during this transitional stage if you frequently remind yourself that by selecting the foods appropriate for your individual body, you are starting a partnership with nature, and supporting it as it regenerates your body.

As I've said, these are only starter menus. Once you integrate your menu into your daily life, you'll be able to augment it with a wide array of foods, herbs, spices, and teas outlined on your individual Diet Sheets in the next chapter. Take a couple weeks to ease into your menu. You're starting a new way of life, and there's no reason to rush and create stress.

Menus for Type O

SUNDAY

Breakfast
Water with lemon
½ grapefruit
1 poached egg
1 or 2 slices spelt toast
1 cup herbal tea

Lunch
110g meat or fish
2 rice cakes or 1 slice bread
Salad: lettuce, bean sprouts, chicory, celery
Dressing: olive oil and lemon juice
1 cup herbal tea

Dinner
110g lean steak, grilled
Steamed kale, Swiss chard, broccoli, dandelion
Salad: cucumbers, bean sprouts, peas
Dressing: olive oil and lemon juice
1 cup herbal tea

MONDAY

Breakfast
Water with lemon
½ grapefruit
Spelt or whole-grain cereal
1 cup herbal tea

Lunch
110g chicken or fish
Tomato and lettuce
1 slice spelt toast
1 cup herbal tea

Dinner
2 lean lamb chops, or pasta
Salad: lettuce, bean sprouts, chicory
Dressing: olive oil and lemon juice
1 cup herbal tea

TUESDAY

Breakfast
Water with lemon
½ grapefruit
1 or 2 poached eggs
1 cup herbal tea

Lunch
110g turkey or fish
Wedges of lettuce, green vegetables, bean sprouts
1 cup herbal tea

Dinner
¼ chicken, skin removed (grilled, baked,
  or boiled)
Steamed broccoli, asparagus, string beans, peas
Salad: lettuce, cucumbers, bean sprouts
Dressing: olive oil and lemon juice
1 cup herbal tea

WEDNESDAY

Breakfast
Water with lemon
½ grapefruit
Kamut or quinoa cereal
1 cup herbal tea

Lunch
110g meat, fish, or fowl
Lettuce, bean sprouts, cucumber
1 cup herbal tea

Dinner
Salmon steak, baked or grilled
Salad: watercress, tomato, mushrooms,
  chicory, celery, kale, bean sprouts
Dressing: olive oil and lemon juice
1 cup herbal tea

THURSDAY

Breakfast
Water with lemon
½ grapefruit
1 or 2 slices toasted spelt bread
1 cup herbal tea

Lunch
110g fish or poultry
Wedges of lettuce, tomatoes, cucumbers,
  bean sprouts
1 cup herbal tea

Dinner
1 veal chop, lean, grilled
Steamed beetroot leaves, dandelion, asparagus
Salad: spinach, mushrooms
Dressing: olive oil and lemon juice
1 cup herbal tea

FRIDAY

Breakfast
Water with lemon
½ grapefruit
1 or 2 slices toasted spelt bread
1 cup herbal tea

Lunch
110g fish, meat, or fowl
Broccoli and string beans mixed
  with olive oil and garlic

Dinner
1 flounder fillet, baked or grilled
Steamed broccoli
Salad: lettuce, cucumbers, bean sprouts
Dressing: olive oil and lemon juice
1 cup herbal tea

SATURDAY

Breakfast
½ grapefruit
Spelt bread
Millet or spelt cereal
1 cup herbal tea

Lunch
Brown rice
Spelt bread
Salad: lettuce, cucumbers, bean sprouts, tomato
Dressing: olive oil and lemon juice
1 cup herbal tea

Dinner
¼ chicken, skin removed (baked, grilled,
  or boiled)
Steamed spinach, endive, broccoli, kale
Salad: lettuce, celery, cucumbers, bean sprouts
Dressing: olive oil and lemon juice
1 cup herbal tea

Notes

- For a late-night snack (all days), choose either an apple or ½ grapefruit. When having fruit before a meal, always wait 10 minutes before eating your meal.

- If you have diabetes or hypoglycemia, reduce carbohydrates and proteins.

- If you have high cholesterol, stay away from milk and cheese, and cut beef from your diet.

- If you have a subtrait of Type B, reduce your intake of turkey, lamb, beef, and buffalo.

- If you have a subtrait of A, lean toward fish, turkey, and lamb; and reduce meat intake in general.

Menus for Type A

SUNDAY

Breakfast
Water with lemon
1 or 2 slices toasted soy bread with tofu spread
   (mix together 1 Tbsp. tofu, 1 Tbsp. almond
   butter, ¼ tsp. olive oil; optional: add chopped
   onion and fresh parsley)
1 cup herbal tea

Lunch
Brown rice
1 slice toasted soy bread
Salad: lettuce, tomato, celery, watercress,
   cucumber, bean sprouts
Dressing: olive oil and lemon juice
1 cup herbal tea

Dinner
¼ chicken, skin removed (boiled or grilled)
Steamed Swiss chard, dandelion, asparagus
Salad: lettuce, cucumber, celery, bean sprouts,
   tomato, ½ square tofu
Dressing: olive oil and lemon juice
1 cup herbal tea

MONDAY

Breakfast
Water with lemon
Millet cereal
1 cup herbal tea

Lunch
Brown rice
Salad: lettuce, stalk of celery, tomato,
½ square tofu, parsley
Dressing: olive oil and lemon juice
1 cup herbal tea

Dinner
1 salmon steak, grilled
Steamed kale, string beans, broccoli tips
Salad: lettuce, tomato, bean sprouts
Dressing: olive oil and lemon juice
1 cup herbal tea

TUESDAY

Breakfast
Water with lemon
1 or 2 slices toasted Kamut bread
(or Ezekiel 4:9 brand of bread) with tofu spread
1 cup herbal tea

Lunch
1 grapefruit
Salad: string beans, cold broccoli
Ezekiel bread
1 cup herbal tea

Dinner
Turkey, skin removed (boiled or grilled)
Steamed dandelion, broccoli tips, asparagus
Salad: lettuce, cucumber, celery, parsley
Dressing: olive oil and lemon juice
1 cup herbal tea

WEDNESDAY

Breakfast
Water with lemon
1 or 2 slices toasted Ezekiel or Kamut bread
with tofu spread
1 cup herbal tea

Lunch
1 can water-packed sardines
Assorted vegetables
Salad: mixed green salad
Dressing: olive oil and lemon juice
1 cup herbal tea

Dinner
½ grapefruit
1 or 2 slices soy or Ezekiel bread
Salad: lettuce, celery, tomato, cucumber,
parsley, spinach, chicory, fresh mushrooms,
½ square tofu
Dressing: olive oil and lemon juice
1 cup herbal tea

THURSDAY

Breakfast
Water with lemon
1 or 2 slices toasted Ezekiel or Kamut bread
with tofu spread
1 cup herbal tea

Lunch
2 hard-boiled eggs
Salad: mixed green salad
Dressing: olive oil and lemon juice
1 cup herbal tea

Dinner
110g grouper, grilled
Steamed string beans
Salad: lettuce, bean sprouts, celery, cucumbers
Dressing: olive oil and lemon juice
1 cup herbal tea

FRIDAY

Breakfast
Water with lemon
1 or 2 slices Ezekiel, spelt, or Kamut bread
  (or cereal)
1 cup herbal tea

Lunch
Salad: lettuce, cucumber, watercress, bean sprouts,
  celery, tomato, ½ square tofu, parsley
Dressing: olive oil and lemon juice
1 cup herbal tea

Dinner
Steamed kale, kelp, okra, Swiss chard, mangetout
Brown rice
Salad: lettuce, celery, chicory, watercress,
  bean sprouts, parsley
Dressing: olive oil and lemon juice
1 slice soy toast
1 cup herbal tea

SATURDAY

Breakfast
Water with lemon
1 or 2 slices toasted Ezekiel bread with tofu spread
1 cup herbal tea

Lunch
Salad: Mix string beans, broccoli, and asparagus
  with scrambled egg whites and tofu
1 slice toasted soy bread
1 cup herbal tea

Dinner
110g haddock, halibut, sole, or salmon
Steamed vegetables
Salad: lettuce, tomato, chicory, celery,
  bean sprouts, cucumber, parsley
Dressing: olive oil and lemon juice
1 cup herbal tea

Notes

- When eating fruit before a meal, always wait 10 minutes before starting your meal.

- If you are diabetic, reduce carbohydrates and proteins.

- If you are hypoglycemic, you crave sugar and starch, but excessive intake will make you tired. Eat protein 3 to 4 times a day in addition to regular meals.

- Although pure Type A's are typically vegetarians, those who have a subtrait of Type A should consider eating fish, lamb, or turkey to ward off fatigue at the beginning of the diet. Reduce meat intake as energy returns.

Menus for Type B

SUNDAY

Breakfast
Water with lemon
½ grapefruit
1 or 2 slices toasted spelt or Ezekiel 4:9 bread with
   tofu spread (mix together 1 Tbsp. tofu, 1 Tbsp.
   almond butter, ¼ tsp. olive oil; optional: add
   chopped onion and fresh parsley)
1 cup herbal tea

Lunch
½ grapefruit
110–170g fish
Mixed greens with asparagus and string beans
Fruit salad made with 1 apple, 1 mango,
   and grapes

Dinner
Turkey (grilled, baked, or boiled)
Steamed beetroot leaves, broccoli, kale
Cucumber salad
Dressing: olive oil and lemon juice
1 cup herbal tea

MONDAY

Breakfast
Water with lemon
½ grapefruit
2 scrambled egg whites and veggies
1 or 2 slices spelt or Ezekiel bread
1 cup herbal tea

Lunch
½ square tofu
Brown rice
Salad: lettuce, bean sprouts, celery, cucumber, chicory, parsley
Dressing: olive oil and lemon juice
1 slice toasted soy bread
1 cup herbal tea

Dinner
1 salmon steak
Steamed string beans, dandelion, broccoli tips
Salad: lettuce, cucumbers, chicory, bean sprouts
Dressing: olive oil and lemon juice
1 cup herbal tea

TUESDAY

Breakfast
Water with lemon
½ grapefruit
1 or 2 slices toasted spelt or Ezekiel bread
    with tofu spread
1 cup herbal tea

Lunch
½ grapefruit
1 slice toasted whole-wheat bread with tofu spread
Mixed green salad
Dressing: olive oil and lemon juice
1 cup herbal tea

Dinner
110–170g lamb, grilled
Steamed beetroot leaves, dandelion, asparagus
Salad: lettuce, bean sprouts, cucumbers
Dressing: olive oil and lemon juice
1 cup herbal tea

WEDNESDAY

Breakfast
Water with lemon
½ grapefruit
Spelt or quinoa cereal
1 cup herbal tea

Lunch
Fruit cocktail made of watermelon, papaya,
　blueberries, blackberries
Mixed green salad
1 cup herbal tea

Dinner
Steamed asparagus and broccoli
Brown rice
Salad: spinach, beetroot leaves, lettuce, chicory,
　mushrooms, tomato, bean sprouts, ½ square tofu
Dressing: olive oil and lemon juice
1 cup herbal tea

THURSDAY

Breakfast
Water with lemon
½ grapefruit
1 or 2 slices toasted spelt or Ezekiel bread
　with tofu spread
1 cup herbal tea

Lunch
2 hard-boiled eggs
Assorted vegetables
Salad: mixed green salad
Dressing: olive oil and lemon juice
1 cup herbal tea

Dinner
1 halibut steak
Steamed kale, endive
Salad: lettuce, cucumbers
Dressing: olive oil and lemon juice
1 cup herbal tea

FRIDAY

Breakfast
Water with lemon
½ grapefruit
Soy or spelt bread
1 cup herbal tea

Lunch
½ square tofu
2 to 3 green vegetables
Salad: lettuce wedges
1 or 2 slices toasted spelt or Ezekiel bread
1 cup herbal tea

Dinner
Turkey, grilled
Steamed broccoli, asparagus
Salad: lettuce, ½ tomato, cucumbers, bean sprouts
Dressing: olive oil and lemon juice
1 cup herbal tea

SATURDAY

Breakfast
Water with lemon
½ grapefruit
1 or 2 eggs
1 cup herbal tea

Lunch
½ square tofu
Brown rice
Salad: spinach with fresh mushrooms
Dressing: olive oil and lemon juice
1 cup herbal tea

Dinner
110–220g lean veal or beef, grilled
Steamed kale, asparagus
Salad: lettuce, tomato, celery, watercress,
   bean sprouts
Dressing: olive oil and lemon juice
1 cup herbal tea

Notes

- When eating fruit before a meal, always wait
  10 minutes before starting your meal.

- For an evening snack, eat an apple once a week; for
  the remainder of days, eat ½ grapefruit.

- If you are Type B with O traits, increase your intake
  of beef.

- If you are Type B with A traits, increase your intake
  of tofu and fish.

- If you are hypoglycemic, increase your protein intake
  by eating a high-protein snack 3 times a day; if you are
  diabetic, decrease your consumption of carbohydrates
  and sugars; and if you have high cholesterol, decrease
  dairy and fatty foods, eat lean meats such as turkey or
  fish, and exercise.

Menus for Type AB

Type AB's should start with the same menu as Type A's. Slowly add small amounts of other foods, such as chicken, fish, whole-wheat products, skimmed milk, and cheeses. By monitoring your responses to these additions, the right levels can be determined. If, for example, nasal congestion develops after adding milk, reduce the amount you're drinking.

Notes

- If you lean toward Type B, increase fish, turkey, and lamb intake. Be sure to exercise.

- If you lean toward Type A, decrease your lamb intake.

- If you are hypoglycemic, reduce carbohydrates and add protein-based snacks such as almonds, sesame or pumpkin seeds, or celery sticks dipped in almond butter 3 times a day. If you are diabetic, avoid carbs. If your cholesterol is elevated, you should try to adopt a vegetarian diet.

I highly recommend that you photocopy or write down your specific menu, and keep it close at hand as you adapt to this new way of eating. I also want to remind you to allow your body to adjust before expanding into the Diet Sheets. The suggested starter menus in this chapter are designed to help you eat high-quality foods and eliminate those that have had a debilitating effect on you. However, your body needs time to get used to this (the time frame is different for everyone depending on your current state of health, but generally takes four to six weeks). For example, if you've been a heavy coffee drinker or have a sweet tooth, you may experience fatigue as a form of withdrawal when you no longer consume caffeine or sugary foods. As you eliminate processed or fast foods laden with preservatives and artificial ingredients, you'll experience a welcome sense of calm.

Start simply, be aware of these physical and mental changes, and gradually move to the more extensive Diet Sheets. As you expand your menu, note how you respond to each new addition. If you feel okay, continue to experiment with different foods. Conversely, if certain foods don't agree with you; for instance, if some raw vegetables in a salad seem to irritate your stomach or cause gas, then cut back or steam them, which may make them easier to digest.

As you explore your new diet, always know that you're following in the footsteps of many of my patients who started their way back to greater health and vitality by taking these same initial steps.

CHAPTER EIGHT

Blood Type and Sub–Blood Type Diet Sheets

Once you've settled into your basic daily menu, you can now expand your diet to include many more meats, fish, vegetables, nuts, herbs, condiments, and herbal teas.

The following Diet Sheets are broken down by blood type and sub–blood type and the frequency in which you can consume various foods per week or month. I've also indicated certain foods that are meant to be eaten once or twice a week; if there is no notation, you may eat these items as often as you wish.

I've created several charts throughout this chapter to help you determine which types of meat and fish would be most beneficial according to your blood type. I've used a numbering system, and the scale ranges from 1 to 3, or as high as 5. For meats, a number 1 means that you can eat it frequently; 2 means several times a week; 3 means once a week; and a 4 or 5 is a food you should eat only on special occasions, such as holidays, celebrations, and when you're dining at someone else's home. Using the example for Type O, you can choose turkey or beef (both are 1's) over chicken (1.5).

Fish is categorized in a similar way, but the numbers indicate the level of toxicity. Using the Type O chart, for example, salmon

(1) and haddock (1.5) would be preferable over halibut (2.5) or sole (3).

All of the foods listed in your specific Diet Sheet can, over time, restore your health and recharge your energy. Please follow this program under the supervision of a qualified physician.

Type-O Diet Sheet

Meat

The numbering of the columns indicates the importance of specific meats in the Type O diet. Number 1 is eaten most often, and number 3 is eaten less often. Meat may be baked or grilled.

1	1.5	2	3
Beef Buffalo Heart (beef or lamb) Ostrich Turkey Veal	Calf's liver* Chicken Lamb	Duck Kidneys (beef or lamb) Partridge Pheasant Quail Rabbit Venison	Beef liver

* Health-food-store purchase only

Fish

Numbering is based on toxicity according to blood type. Number 1 is the least toxic, and 4 is the most toxic. Farm-raised fish is not desirable; wild is preferred. Fish may be baked, grilled, or boiled (do not fry).

1	1.5	2	2.5	3	4
Salmon	Arctic char Cod (Dec.–Apr.) Haddock Orange roughy	Grouper Kingfish Mahimahi Monkfish Sardines* Scrod Shad Skate Trout Turbot Whitefish	Halibut	Bass Flounder Pike Sole	Hake Mackerel Red snapper Sturgeon Tilapia

* In water

Type O's should consume a total of 14 to 16 servings per week of meat and fish.

Eggs

Type O's can eat five whole eggs per week with vegetables. Free-range eggs are preferred. Do not fry.

Cheese

Look for cheeses that don't contain food coloring, additives, or preservatives.

Feta**
Goat*
Manchego** (or similar cheeses)
Mozzarella**
Ricotta**

Occasionally (once per week)
**Rarely (once per month)*

Cereals

Amaranth	Puffed rice
Brown rice cream	Quinoa
Kamut	Rice bran
Millet	Spelt
Oat bran*	Sprouted grain cereal
Oatmeal*	

Occasionally (once per week)

Milk for Cereals
(Unsweetened)

Almond milk
Rice milk
Soy milk**

** *Rarely (once per month)*

Bread and Crackers
(Yeast Free)

Almond	Rice
Essene	Rice cakes
Ezekiel	Spelt
Kamut	Sprouted wheat
Quinoa	

Pasta	*or*	**Grains**
Rice		Amaranth
Soy		Barley
Spelt		Basmati rice
		Brown rice
		Buckwheat (kasha)
		Bulgur
		Millet
		Quinoa
		Spelt
		Teff
		Wild rice

Starchy Vegetables

Jerusalem artichokes
Potatoes (white, blue, and red)
Sweet potatoes

Dried Peas, Beans, and Lentils
(Legume Family)

Cannellini**
Chickpeas**
Fava**
Kidney**
Lentil**

** *Rarely (once per month)*

Vegetables
(Fresh or Frozen)

Artichokes
Asparagus
Bamboo shoots
Beetroot leaves
Beetroot (small)
Belgian endive
Broccoli (with lemon)
Brussels sprouts**
Cabbage (white)*
Capers
Carrots (raw or boiled)
Cauliflower*
Celery
Celery root
Chicory
Chinese cabbage
Collards*
Courgette
Cucumber
Daikon

Dandelion greens
Dill
Endive
Fiddleheads
Garlic clove
Green onion
Jerusalem artichoke (fresh)
Jicama
Kale
Kohlrabi
Leek
Lettuce (all types)
Okra
Mangetout
Olives (green)
Onions
Parsley
Parsnips
Peas
Peppers (green, red, or hot)

Radishes
Rapini
Rocket
Savoy cabbage
Seaweed (all types)
Shallots
Shiitake mushrooms
Spinach (raw)
Sprouts (all types)
Squash (winter or summer)
String beans (green or yellow)
Swede
Swiss chard
Tomato
Water chestnuts
Watercress

* *Occasionally (once per week)*
** *Rarely (once per month)*

For a wonderful vegetable soup, try the Vegetarian Soup recipe in Chapter 11. Make a large quantity so that you can eat a couple of ladles once or twice a day.

Nuts and Seeds

All varieties should be raw, unsalted, and in the shells, if possible; be sure to chew well. (A handful is about 4 Tbsp., or 25g.)

Almonds	Pine nuts
Brazil nuts	Pistachios*
Chestnuts*	Pumpkin seeds
Flaxseeds	Sesame seeds**
Hazelnuts	Sunflower seeds
Pecans	Walnuts

Occasionally (once per week)
**Rarely (once per month)*

Nut and Seed Butters

All varieties should be raw, smooth, and without sugar or additives.

Almond
Macadamia
Sunflower

Fruits
(Fresh only or dried where indicated)

Acid	Subacid	Sweet	Neutral
Cranberries	Apples	Currants (black)	Breadfruit
Grapefruit	Apricots	Dates	Star apples
Lemons	Blackberries	Figs (dried)	Watermelon
Limes	Blueberries	Kumquats	
Pineapples	Cherries	Persimmons	
Pomegranates	Figs (fresh)	Prunes*	
Raspberries	Gooseberries	Raisins (red)	
Strawberries	Grapes (blue)		
	Kiwi		
	Loganberries		
	Mangoes		
	Nectarines		
	Papayas		
	Peaches		
	Pears		
	Plums (dark)		

* Occasionally (once per week)

Lemons may be eaten as often as you desire and may be combined with any food. Strawberries should always be eaten alone.

Juices

Juice should be freshly squeezed and kept in glass jars, or bought frozen and unsweetened. Type O's can have 480ml to 1.2L per day total; each serving should contain ¼ juice and ¾ springwater.

Apple	Cherry	Papaya
Apricot	Cranberry	Peach
Black cherry	Grape	Pineapple
Blueberry	Grapefruit	Prune**
Carrot	Lemon and water	Tomato
Celery	Nectarine	

** Rarely (once per month)

Saturated and Unsaturated Fats

All oils should be cold-pressed, preferably organic, and contain no genetically modified ingredients. Don't use olive oil for cooking, as when the oil is heated, its molecular composition changes. It loses its full nutritional value and can even be carcinogenic. Grape-seed oil has a higher tolerance to heat and should be used instead.

Flaxseed oil
Grape-seed oil
Olive oil
Safflower oil*
Sesame oil*
Sunflower oil*

* Occasionally (once per week)

The D'Adamo Institute created a healthy spread (the Institute's Spread) that can be used in place of margarine or pure butter. Type O's should use ¼ teaspoon three times per week.

Institute's Spread

110g sweet butter
60ml grape-seed or olive oil
1 vitamin E capsule
1 lecithin capsule

Whip ingredients together and refrigerate.

Herbs

Basil	Fennel	Rosemary
Bay leaf	Garlic clove	Sage
Celery seed	Lemongrass	Savory
Chervil	Marjoram	Spring onion
Chives	Mint	Tarragon
Coriander	Oregano	Thyme
Dill	Parsley	

Spices

Anise	Coriander	Mustard seed
Caraway	Cumin	Nutmeg
Cayenne	Curry powder	Paprika**
Chilli pepper	Fenugreek	Saffron
Cinnamon	Ginger	Turmeric
Cloves	Mustard (dried)	

*** Rarely (once per month)*

Condiments

Dulse flakes	Unprocessed apple-cider vinegar
Kelp powder	Vegetable salt
Pure vanilla bean	Wheat-free tamari
Sea salt	

Herbal Teas

These teas have individual therapeutic values and are very beneficial. You may drink them as often as desired. Prepare teas with springwater or reverse-osmosis water. Measure 1 tsp. of herb tea into 235ml of boiled water, and allow it to stand 5 to 6 minutes. Never add sugar, milk, or lemon.

Alfalfa	Ginseng (instant)	Nettle
Avena sativa	Ginseng root	Parsley
Barley	Ginseng (Siberian)	Peppermint
Basil leaf	Goldenseal	Raspberry
Burdock	Hawthorn	Rose hip
Caraway seed	Holy thistle	Saint-John's-wort
Chamomile	Horsetail	Skullcap
Chickweed	Japanese green tea	Slippery elm
Corn silk	Juniper	Solomon's seal
Dandelion leaves	Lady's mantle	Strawberry
Dill seed	Liquorice root	Tanacetum
Fenugreek	Linden	Uva-ursi
Fern	Marshmallow	White birch
Fig	Maté	White tea
Ginger	Mistletoe	

Morning Routine

Upon rising, squeeze ¼ or ½ fresh lemon into 100ml of cold water.

Type-O Energy Drink

1 Tbsp. whey protein powder
1 tsp. psyllium powder
1 tsp. stractan
1 tsp. flaxseed oil

Mix ingredients in 175 to 235ml of water, diluted grapefruit juice, or soy (or rice) milk. Drink one to three times daily.

Type-Oa Diet Sheet

Meat

The numbering of the columns indicates the importance of specific meats in the Type Oa diet. Number 1 is eaten most often, and number 3 is eaten less often. Meat may be baked or grilled.

1	1.5	2	3
Ostrich Turkey	Chicken	Buffalo Duck Lamb	Beef Rabbit Veal Venison

Fish

Numbering is based on toxicity according to blood type. Number 1 is the least toxic, and 4 is the most toxic. Farm-raised fish is not desirable; wild is preferred. Fish may be baked, grilled, or boiled (do not fry).

1	1.5	2	2.5	3	4
Salmon	Arctic char Cod (Dec.–Apr.) Haddock Orange roughy	Grouper Kingfish Scrod Skate Trout Turbot	Whitefish	Bass Flounder Halibut Mahimahi Sardines*	Hake Red snapper Sole Sturgeon Tilapia

* In water

Type Oa's should consume a total of 7 to 9 servings per week of meat and fish.

Eggs

Type Oa's can consume three eggs per week. Free-range eggs are preferred. Eat them with vegetables and occasionally, tofu; alternatively, make an egg-white omelette with tofu and vegetables (such as broccoli and asparagus). Don't use store-bought egg whites. Egg whites may be poached, scrambled, or hard-boiled; do not fry.

Cereals

Amaranth	Quinoa
Brown rice cereal	Rice bran
Kamut	Spelt
Puffed rice	Sprouted grain cereal

Milk for Cereals
(Unsweetened)

Almond milk*
Rice milk
Soy milk*

Occasionally (once per week)

Bread and Crackers

Essene	Rice cakes
Ezekiel (yeast free)	Soya
Kamut	Spelt*
Quinoa	Sprouted wheat

Occasionally (once per week)

Pasta	*or*	**Grains**
Artichoke		Amaranth
Rice		Barley
Soy*		Basmati rice
Spelt		Brown rice
		Buckwheat (kasha)*
		Bulgur
		Millet
		Quinoa
		Spelt*
		Teff
		Wild rice

* Occasionally (once per week)

Starchy Vegetables

Jerusalem artichokes
Potatoes (white, blue, and red)
Sweet potatoes

Dried Peas, Beans, and Lentils
(Legume Family)

Adzuki**
Cannellini**
Chickpeas**
Fava**
Kidney**
Lentil**
Soy**

** Rarely (once per month)

Vegetables
(Fresh or Frozen)

Artichokes
Asparagus
Bamboo shoots
Beetroot leaves
Beetroot (small)
Belgian endive
Broccoli (with lemon)
Brussels sprouts**
Capers
Carrots (boiled and raw**)
Cauliflower**
Celery
Celery root
Chicory
Chinese cabbage
Courgette
Daikon
Dandelion greens

Dill
Endive
Fiddleheads
Garlic clove
Green onion
Jerusalem artichokes (fresh)
Jicama
Kale
Kohlrabi
Leeks
Lettuce (all types)
Mangetout
Mushrooms**
Okra
Olives (green)
Onions
Parsley
Peas
Peppers (green*,

hot*, and red)
Radishes
Rapini
Rocket
Seaweed (all types)
Shallots
Shiitake mushrooms
Soybeans (fresh)*
Spinach (raw)
Sprouts (all types)
String beans (green and yellow)
Squash (summer and winter)
Swiss chard
Tomato*
Water chestnuts
Watercress

Occasionally (once per week)
**Rarely (once per month)*

For a wonderful vegetable soup, try the Vegetarian Soup recipe in Chapter 11. Type Oa's can eat this one to seven times per week.

Nuts and Seeds

All varieties should be raw, unsalted, and in the shells, if possible; be sure to chew well. (A handful is about 4 Tbsp., or 25g.)

Almonds	Pine nuts
Brazil nuts	Pumpkin seeds
Chestnuts*	Sesame seeds*
Flaxseeds	Sunflower seeds
Pecans	Walnuts

* Occasionally (once per week)

Nut and Seed Butters

All varieties should be raw, smooth, and without sugar or additives.

Almond
Macadamia
Soy**
Sunflower
Tahini (sesame butter)*

* Occasionally (once per week)
** Rarely (once per month)

Fruits
(Fresh only)

Acid	Subacid	Sweet	Neutral
Cranberries	Apricots	Dates	Breadfruit
Grapefruit	Blackberries	Kumquats	Star apples
Lemons	Blueberries	Persimmons	Watermelon
Limes	Cherries	Pomegranates	
Pineapples	Figs	Raisins (red)	
Pomegranates	Gooseberries		
Raspberries	Grapes (blue)		
Strawberries	Kiwi		
	Loganberries		
	Mangoes		
	Nectarines		
	Papayas		
	Peaches		
	Pears		
	Plums (dark)		

Lemons may be eaten as often as you desire and may be combined with any food. Strawberries should always be eaten alone.

Juices

Juice should be freshly squeezed and kept in glass jars, or bought frozen and unsweetened. Type Oa's can have 480ml to 1.5L per day total; each serving should contain ¼ juice and ¾ springwater.

Apricot	Grapefruit
Black cherry	Lemon and water
Blueberry	Nectarine
Celery	Papaya
Cranberry	Pineapple
Grape	

Saturated and Unsaturated Fat

All oils should be cold-pressed, preferably organic, and contain no genetically modified ingredients. Don't use olive oil for cooking, as when the oil is heated, its molecular composition changes. It loses its full nutritional value and can even be carcinogenic. Grape-seed oil has a higher tolerance to heat and should be used instead.

Flaxseed oil	Safflower oil*
Grape-seed oil	Sesame oil*
Olive oil	Soy oil*
Peanut oil*	Sunflower oil*

* Occasionally (once per week)

The D'Adamo Institute created a healthy spread (the Institute's Spread) that can be used in place of margarine or pure butter. Type Oa's should use ¼ teaspoon two times per week.

Institute's Spread

110g sweet butter
60ml grape-seed or olive oil
1 vitamin E capsule
1 lecithin capsule

Whip ingredients together and refrigerate.

Herbs

Basil	Fennel	Sage
Bay leaf	Garlic clove	Savory
Celery seed	Lemongrass	Spring Onion
Chervil	Mint	Tarragon
Chives	Oregano	Thyme
Coriander	Parsley	
Dill	Rosemary	

Spices

Anise	Coriander	Mustard seed*
Caraway	Cumin	Nutmeg*
Cayenne*	Fenugreek	Saffron*
Cinnamon	Ginger	Turmeric
Cloves	Mustard (dried)	

Occasionally (once per week)

Condiments

Dulse flakes	Sea salt
Kelp powder	Vegetable salt
Miso**	Wheat-free tamari
Pure vanilla bean	

** *Rarely (once per month)*

Herbal Teas

These teas have individual therapeutic values and are very beneficial. You may drink them as often as desired. Prepare teas with springwater or reverse-osmosis water. Measure 1 tsp. of herb tea into 235ml of boiled water, and allow it to stand 5 to 6 minutes. Never add sugar, milk, or lemon.

Alfalfa	Goldenseal	Parsley
Avena sativa	Hawthorn	Peppermint
Chamomile	Holy thistle*	Raspberry
Chickweed	Horsetail	Rose hip*
Corn silk	Japanese green tea	Saint-John's-wort*
Dandelion leaves	Juniper	Skullcap
Fenugreek	Liquorice root	Slippery elm
Fern	Linden	Tanacetum
Ginger	Marshmallow	Uva-ursi
Ginseng (instant)	Maté*	White tea
Ginseng root	Mistletoe	
Ginseng (Siberian)	Nettle	

* Occasionally (once per week)

Morning Routine

Upon rising, squeeze ¼ or ½ fresh lemon into 3½ oz. of cool water.

Type-Oa Energy Drink

1 Tbsp. soy (or whey) protein powder
1 tsp. psyllium powder
1 tsp. stractan

Mix ingredients in 175ml to 235ml of water, diluted grapefruit juice, or soy (or rice) milk. Drink one to three times daily.

Type-Ob Diet Sheet

Meat

The numbering of the columns indicates the importance of specific meats in the Type Ob diet. Number 1 is eaten most often, and number 4 is eaten less often. Meat may be baked or grilled.

1	1.5	2	3	4
Buffalo Lamb Ostrich Turkey	Calf's liver*	Beef Duck Quail Rabbit Venison	Chicken Veal	Beef liver

* Health-food-store purchase only

Fish

Numbering is based on toxicity according to blood type. Number 1 is the least toxic, and 4 is the most toxic. Farm-raised fish is not desirable; wild is preferred. Fish may be baked, grilled, or boiled (do not fry).

1	1.5	2	2.5	3	4
Salmon	Arctic char Cod (Dec.–Apr.) Haddock Orange roughy	Grouper Kingfish Mahimahi Scrod Shad Skate Trout Turbot	Monkfish Sturgeon Whitefish	Bass Flounder Halibut Sardines* Sole	Hake Mackerel Red snapper Tilapia

* In water

Type Ob's should consume a total of 12 to 15 servings per week of meat and fish.

Eggs

Type Ob's can eat three to four whole eggs per week with vegetables. Free-range eggs are preferred. Do not fry.

Cheese

Type Ob's should consume 170g of cheese per week. Look for
cheeses that don't contain food coloring, additives, or preservatives.

Goat's cheese
Mozzarella
Ricotta

Milk Products
(120ml per week)

Goat's milk
Yogurt, plain (whole milk or 2 percent)

Cereals

Amaranth	Puffed rice
Brown rice cereal	Quinoa
Kamut	Rice bran
Millet	Spelt
Oat bran*	Sprouted grain cereal
Oatmeal*	

* Occasionally (once per week)

Milk for Cereals
(Unsweetened)

Almond milk
Oat milk
Rice milk

Bread and Crackers

Almond
Essene
Ezekiel
Kamut
Quinoa

Rice
Rice cakes
Spelt
Sprouted wheat

Pasta (110g or less)   *or*   **Grains**
Artichoke   Amaranth
Rice   Barley
Spelt   Basmati rice
                               Brown rice
                               Buckwheat (kasha)*
                               Bulgur
                               Millet
                               Quinoa
                               Spelt
                               Teff
                               Wild rice

Occasionally (once per week)

Starchy Vegetables

Jerusalem artichokes
Potatoes (white, blue, and red)
Sweet potatoes

Dried Peas, Beans, and Lentils
(Legume Family)

Adzuki**
Cannellini**
Chickpeas**
Fava**
Kidney**
Lentil**

** *Rarely (once per month)*

Vegetables
(Fresh or Frozen)

Artichokes
Asparagus
Bamboo shoots
Beetroot leaves
Beetroot (small)
Belgian endive
Broccoli
(with lemon)
Brussels sprouts*
Cabbage
(white** or red**)
Carrots (raw or
boiled*)
Cauliflower**
Celery
Celery root
Chicory
Chinese cabbage*
Collards*
Courgettes
Cucumber
Daikon

Dandelion greens
Dill
Endive
Fiddleheads
Garlic clove
Green onion
Jerusalem
artichoke (fresh)
Jicama
Kale
Kohlrabi
Leek
Lettuce (all types)
Mangetout
Mushrooms
Mustard greens
Okra
Olives (green)
Onions
Parsley
Peas
Peppers (green, red,

or hot*)
Radishes
Rapini
Rocket
Savoy cabbage*
Seaweed (all types)
Shallots
Shiitake
mushrooms
Spinach (raw)
Spring onion
Sprouts (all types)
Squash (winter
or summer)
String beans (green
or yellow)
Swiss chard
Swede
Tomato*
Water chestnuts*
Watercress

* *Occasionally (once per week)*
** *Rarely (once per month)*

Nuts and Seeds

All varieties should be raw, unsalted, and in the shells, if possible; be sure to chew well. (A handful is about 4 Tbsp., or 60g.)

Almonds	Pine nuts
Brazil nuts	Pistachios*
Chestnuts*	Pumpkin seeds
Flaxseeds	Sesame seeds**
Hazelnuts	Sunflower seeds
Pecans	Walnuts

Occasionally (once per week)
**Rarely (once per month)*

Nut and Seed Butters

All varieties should be raw, smooth, and without sugar or additives.

Almond
Macadamia
Sunflower
Tahini (sesame butter)

Tofu

Use organic tofu and eat it rarely (once per month).

Fruits
(Fresh only or dried where indicated)

Acid	Subacid	Sweet	Neutral
Cranberries	Apples	Currants (black)	Breadfruit
Grapefruit	Apricots	Dates	Star apples
Lemons	Blackberries	Figs (dried)	Watermelon
Limes	Blueberries	Kumquats	
Pineapples	Cherries	Persimmons	
Pomegranates	Figs (fresh)	Pomegranates	
Raspberries	Gooseberries	Prunes*	
Strawberries	Grapes (blue)	Raisins (red)	
	Kiwi		
	Loganberries		
	Mangoes		
	Nectarines		
	Papayas		
	Peaches		
	Pears		
	Plums (dark)		

Occasionally (once per week)

Lemons may be eaten as often as you desire and may be combined with any food. Strawberries should always be eaten alone.

Juices

Juice should be freshly squeezed and kept in glass jars, or bought frozen and unsweetened. Type Ob's can have 480ml to 1.5L per day total; each serving should contain ¼ juice and ¾ springwater.

Apple	Cherry	Papaya
Apricot	Cranberry	Pineapple
Black cherry	Grape	Prune*
Blueberry	Grapefruit	Tomato**
Carrot	Lemon and water	
Celery	Nectarine	

Occasionally (once per week)
**Rarely (once per month)*

Saturated and Unsaturated Fats

All oils should be cold-pressed, preferably organic, and contain no genetically modified ingredients. Don't use olive oil for cooking, as when the oil is heated, its molecular composition changes. It loses its full nutritional value and can even be carcinogenic. Grape-seed oil has a higher tolerance to heat and should be used instead.

Flaxseed oil	Safflower oil*
Grape-seed oil	Sesame oil*
Olive oil	Sunflower oil*

* Occasionally (once per week)

The D'Adamo Institute created a healthy spread (the Institute's Spread) that can be used in place of margarine or pure butter. Type Ob's should use ⅛ teaspoon three times per week.

Institute's Spread

110g sweet butter
60ml grape-seed or olive oil
1 vitamin E capsule
1 lecithin capsule

Whip ingredients together and refrigerate.

Herbs

Basil	Fennel	Rosemary
Bay leaf	Garlic clove	Sage
Celery seed	Lemongrass	Savory
Chervil	Marjoram	Spring onions
Chives	Mint	Tarragon
Coriander	Oregano	Thyme
Dill	Parsley	

Spices

Anise	Coriander	Mustard seed*
Caraway	Cumin	Nutmeg*
Cayenne	Curry powder	Paprika*
Chilli pepper	Fenugreek	Saffron
Cinnamon	Ginger	Turmeric
Cloves	Mustard (dried)	

* Occasionally (once per week)

Condiments

Dulse flakes	Unprocessed apple-cider vinegar*
Kelp powder	
Miso**	Vegetable salt
Sea salt	Wheat-free tamari

* Occasionally (once per week)
** Rarely (once per month)

Herbal Teas

These teas have individual therapeutic values and are very beneficial. You may drink them as often as desired. Prepare teas with springwater or reverse-osmosis water. Measure 1 tsp. of herb tea into 235ml of boiled water, and allow it to stand 5 to 6 minutes. Never add sugar, milk, or lemon.

Alfalfa	Ginseng root	Parsley
Avena sativa	Goldenseal	Peppermint
Barley	Hawthorn	Raspberry
Basil leaf	Holy thistle	Rose hip
Caraway seed	Horsetail	Saint-John's-wort
Chamomile	Japanese green tea	Skullcap
Chickweed	Juniper	Slippery elm
Corn silk	Lady's mantle	Solomon's seal
Dandelion leaves	Liquorice root	Strawberry
Dill seed	Linden	Tanacetum
Fenugreek	Marshmallow	Uva-ursi
Fern	Maté	White birch
Ginger	Mistletoe	White tea
Ginseng (instant)	Nettle	

Morning Routine

Upon rising, squeeze ¼ or ½ fresh lemon into 100ml of cool to cold water.

Type-Ob Energy Drink

1 Tbsp. soy or whey protein powder
1 tsp. psyllium powder
1 tsp. stractan
1 tsp. flaxseed oil

Mix ingredients in 175 to 235ml of water, diluted grapefruit juice, or soy (or rice) milk. Drink one to three times daily.

Type-A Diet Sheet

Fish

Numbering is based on toxicity according to blood type. Number 1 is the least toxic, and 4 is the most toxic. Farm-raised fish is not desirable; wild is preferred. Fish may be baked, grilled, or boiled (do not fry). Type A's can eat fish two to three times per week.

1	1.5	2	3	4
Salmon	Arctic char Cod (Dec.–Apr.) Haddock Orange roughy	Grouper Kingfish Skate Trout Turbot	Bass Flounder Halibut Mahimahi Scrod Sole Sturgeon Whitefish	Hake Red snapper Tilapia

Eggs

Type A's can eat two eggs per week with tofu or vegetables. Use egg whites only (don't use store-bought egg whites). Free-range eggs are preferred. Eggs may be poached, scrambled, or hard-boiled. Do not fry.

Starch

Avoid products that contain wheat.

Cereals

Cereals may be eaten with unsweetened soy milk.

Amaranth   Quinoa
Brown rice cereal   Rice bran
Kamut   Spelt
Puffed rice   Sprouted grain cereal

Bread and Crackers
(Yeast Free)

Almond   Rice
Essene   Soy
Ezekiel (without yeast)   Sprouted wheat
Kamut

Pasta   *or*   **Grains**
Artichoke   Amaranth
Rice   Barley
Soy   Basmati rice
Spelt   Brown rice
                             Buckwheat (kasha)*
                             Bulgur
                             Millet
                             Quinoa
                             Spelt*
                             Teff
                             Wild rice

* Occasionally (once per week)

Starchy Vegetables
(Baked)

Jerusalem artichokes
Potatoes (white, blue, and red)
Pumpkin
Sweet potatoes
Yams

Dried Peas, Beans, and Lentils
(Legume Family)

Adzuki*
Cannellini*
Chickpeas*
Fava*
Lentils*
Soy

Occasionally (once per week)

Vegetables
(Fresh or Frozen)

Artichokes

Asparagus

Bamboo shoots

Beetroot leaves

Beetroots (small)

Belgian endive

Broccoli
(with lemon)

Brussels sprouts*

Carrots (boiled)

Celery

Celery root

Chicory

Chinese cabbage

Courgettes

Daikon

Dandelion greens

Dill

Endive

Fiddleheads

Garlic clove

Green onion

Jerusalem
artichoke (fresh)

Jicama

Kale

Kohlrabi

Leeks

Lettuce (all types)

Mangetout

Okra

Olives (green)**

Onions

Parsley

Peas

Peppers
(green* or red*)

Rapini*

Rocket

Savoy cabbage**

Seaweed (all types)

Shallots

Shiitake
mushrooms*

Soy beans (fresh)

Spinach (raw)**

Spring onions

Sprouts (all types)

Squash (winter
or summer)

String beans
(green or yellow)

Swiss chard

Tomato**

Water chestnuts

Watercress

Occasionally (once per week)
**Rarely (once per month)*

For a wonderful vegetable soup, try the Vegetarian Soup recipe in Chapter 11. Type A's should have this soup one to seven times per week.

Nuts and Seeds

All varieties should be raw, unsalted, and in the shells, if possible; be sure to chew well. (A handful is about 4 Tbsp., or 60g.)

Almonds	Pine nuts
Brazil nuts	Pumpkin seeds
Chestnuts*	Sesame seeds*
Flaxseeds	Sunflower seeds
Pecans	Walnuts

Occasionally (once per week)

Nut and Seed Butters

All varieties should be raw, smooth, and without sugar or additives. Have one to two Tbsp. per day on rice cakes, crackers, or celery sticks.

Almond
Macadamia
Soy
Sunflower*
Tahini (sesame butter)*

Occasionally (once per week)

Tofu

Tofu is a good source of vegetable protein. Type A's should have at least seven servings of organic tofu per week.

Fruits
(Fresh only or dried where indicated)

Acid	Subacid	Sweet	Neutral
Cranberries	Apricots	Dates	Breadfruit
Grapefruit	Blackberries	Figs (dried)	Star apples
Lemons	Blueberries	Kumquats	Watermelon
Limes	Figs (fresh)	Persimmons	
Pineapples	Gooseberries	Raisins (red)	
Pomegranates	Grapes (blue)		
Raspberries	Kiwi		
Strawberries	Loganberries		
	Mangoes		
	Nectarines		
	Papayas		
	Peaches		
	Pears		
	Plums (dark)		

Lemons may be eaten as often as you desire and may be combined with any food. Strawberries should always be eaten alone.

Juices

Juice should be freshly squeezed and kept in glass jars, or bought frozen and unsweetened. Type A's can have 480ml to 1.5L per day; each serving should contain ¼ juice and ¾ springwater.

Apricot	Cranberry	Nectarine
Black cherry	Grape	Papaya
Blueberry	Grapefruit	Pineapple
Celery	Lemon and water	

Saturated and Unsaturated Fats

All oils should be cold-pressed, preferably organic, and contain no genetically modified ingredients. Don't use olive oil for cooking, as when the oil is heated, its molecular composition changes. It loses its full nutritional value and can even be carcinogenic. Grape-seed oil has a higher tolerance to heat and should be used instead.

Flaxseed oil	Safflower oil*
Grape-seed oil	Sesame oil*
Olive oil	Soy oil*
Peanut oil*	Sunflower oil*

* Occasionally (once per week)

Herbs

Basil	Fennel	Sage
Bay leaf	Garlic clove	Savory
Celery seed	Lemongrass	Spring onion
Chervil	Mint	Tarragon
Chives	Oregano	Thyme
Coriander	Parsley	
Dill	Rosemary	

Spices

Anise	Fenugreek	Saffron*
Cinnamon	Ginger	Turmeric
Coriander	Mustard (dried)*	
Cumin	Mustard seed*	

* Occasionally (once per week)

Condiments

Dulse flakes

Kelp powder

Miso

Pure vanilla bean*

Sea salt

Tempeh*

Vegetable salt

Wheat-free tamari

* Occasionally (once per week)

Herbal Teas

These teas have individual therapeutic values and are very beneficial. You may drink them as often as desired. Prepare teas with springwater or reverse-osmosis water. Measure 1 tsp. of herb tea into 235ml of boiled water, and allow it to stand 5 to 6 minutes. Never add sugar, milk, or lemon.

Alfalfa	Ginseng (instant)	Nettle
Avena sativa	Ginseng root	Parsley
Basil leaf	Ginseng (Siberian)	Peppermint
Chamomile	Goldenseal	Rose hip*
Chickweed	Hawthorn	Saint-John's-wort
Corn silk	Horsetail	Skullcap
Dandelion leaves	Japanese green tea	Slippery elm
Fenugreek	Juniper	Uva-ursi
Fern	Linden	White tea
Ginger	Marshmallow	

* Occasionally (once per week)

Morning Routine

Upon rising, squeeze ¼ fresh lemon into 3 oz. of warm water.

Type-A Energy Drink

1 Tbsp. soy protein powder
1 tsp. psyllium powder
1 tsp. stractan

Mix ingredients in 175 to 235ml of water, diluted grapefruit juice, or soy (or rice) milk. Drink one to three times daily.

Type-Ab Diet Sheet

If you're perfectly healthy, you should adopt a vegetarian diet. If, however, you feel some fatigue, add fish; if you're often fatigued, add turkey to your diet.

Meat

The numbering of the columns indicates the importance of specific meats in the Type Ab diet. Number 1 is eaten most often, and number 4 is eaten less often. Meat may be baked or grilled.

1	1.5	2	3	3.5	4
Turkey	Lamb Ostrich	Buffalo	Duck	Chicken	Beef

Fish

Numbering is based on toxicity according to blood type. Number 1 is the least toxic, and 4 is the most toxic. Farm-raised fish is not desirable; wild is preferred. Fish may be baked, grilled, or boiled (do not fry).

1	1.5	2	2.5	3	4
Salmon	Arctic char Cod (Dec.–Apr.) Haddock Orange roughy	Grouper Kingfish Scrod Skate Trout Turbot	Whitefish	Bass Flounder Halibut Mahimahi	Hake Red snapper Sole Sturgeon Tilapia

Type Ab's should consume a total of 5 to 7 servings per week of meat and fish.

Eggs

Type Ab's can consume three egg whites per week with vegetables or tofu. Do not use store-bought egg whites; free-range eggs are preferable. Egg whites may be poached, scrambled, or boiled; do not fry.

Cheese

Look for cheeses that don't contain food coloring, additives, or preservatives.

Feta**
Mozzarella**
Ricotta**

** *Rarely (once per month)*

Starches

Avoid products that contain wheat.

Cereals

Amaranth	Quinoa
Brown rice cereal	Rice bran
Kamut	Spelt
Puffed rice	Sprouted grain cereal

Milk for Cereals
(Unsweetened)

Rice milk*
Soy milk

* *Occasionally (once per week)*

Bread and Crackers
(Yeast Free)

Essene
Ezekiel
Soy

Pasta	*or*	**Grains**
Artichoke		Amaranth
Rice		Basmati rice
Soy		Brown rice
Spelt		Buckwheat (kasha)*
		Bulgur
		Millet
		Quinoa
		Spelt*
		Teff
		Wild rice

* *Occasionally (once per week)*

Starchy Vegetables
(Baked)

Jerusalem artichokes
Potatoes (white, blue, and red)
Sweet potatoes
Yams

Dried Peas, Beans, and Lentils
(Legume Family)

Adzuki*
Cannellini**
Chickpeas
Fava**

Occasionally (once per week)
**Rarely (once per month)*

Vegetables
(Fresh or Frozen)

Artichokes
Asparagus
Bamboo shoots
Beetroot leaves
Beetroot (small)
Belgian endive
Broccoli
(with lemon)
Brussels sprouts*
Carrots (boiled)
Celery
Celery root
Chicory
Chinese cabbage
Courgettes
Cucumber*
Daikon
Dandelion greens
Dill
Endive

Fiddleheads
Garlic clove
Green onion
Jerusalem
artichoke (fresh)
Jicama
Kale
Kohlrabi
Leeks
Lettuce (all types)
Mangetout
Mushrooms*
Okra
Olives (green)
Onions
Parsley
Peas
Peppers (green,
red, or hot**)
Radishes*

Rapini
Rocket
Savoy cabbage*
Spring onions
Seaweed (all types)
Shallots
Shiitake
mushrooms
Soy beans (fresh)
Spinach (raw)
Sprouts (all types)
Squash (winter
or summer)
String beans
(green or yellow)
Swiss chard
Tomato**
Water chestnuts
Watercress

Occasionally (once per week)
**Rarely (once per month)*

Nuts and Seeds

All varieties should be raw, unsalted, and in the shells, if possible; be sure to chew well. (A handful is about 4 Tbsp., or 60g.)

Almonds	Pine nuts
Brazil nuts	Pumpkin seeds
Chestnuts*	Sesame seeds*
Flaxseeds	Sunflower seeds
Pecans	Walnuts

Occasionally (once per week)

Nut and Seed Butters

All varieties should be raw, smooth, and without sugar or additives.

Almond
Macadamia
Soy
Sunflower*
Tahini (sesame butter)*

Occasionally (once per week)

Tofu

Tofu is a good source of vegetable protein. Type Ab's should eat organic tofu three to four times per week.

Fruits
(Fresh only or dried where indicated)

Acid	Subacid	Sweet	Neutral
Cranberries	Apricots	Currants (black)	Breadfruit
Grapefruit	Blackberries	Dates	Star apples
Lemons	Blueberries	Figs (dried)	Watermelon
Limes	Figs (fresh)	Kumquats	
Pineapples	Gooseberries	Pomegranates	
Pomegranates	Grapes (blue)	Raisins (red)	
Raspberries	Guava		
Strawberries	Kiwi		
	Loganberries		
	Mangoes		
	Nectarines		
	Papayas		
	Peaches		
	Pears		
	Plums (dark)		

Lemons may be eaten as often as you desire and may be combined with any food. Strawberries should always be eaten alone.

Juices

Juice should be freshly squeezed and kept in glass jars, or bought frozen and unsweetened. Type Ab's can have 480ml to 1.65L per day; each serving should contain ¼ juice and ¾ springwater.

Apricot	Cranberry	Papaya
Black cherry	Grape	Pineapple
Blueberry	Grapefruit	
Celery	Lemon and water	

Saturated and Unsaturated Fats

All oils should be cold-pressed, preferably organic, and contain no genetically modified ingredients. Don't use olive oil for cooking, as when the oil is heated, its molecular composition changes. It loses its full nutritional value and can even be carcinogenic. Grape-seed oil has a higher tolerance to heat and should be used instead.

Flaxseed oil	Safflower oil*
Grape-seed oil	Sesame oil*
Olive oil	Soy oil*
Peanut oil*	Sunflower oil*

Occasionally (once per week)

Herbs

Basil	Fennel	Sage
Bay leaf	Garlic clove	Savory
Celery seed	Lemongrass	Spring onions
Chervil	Mint	Tarragon
Chives	Oregano	Thyme
Coriander	Parsley	
Dill	Rosemary	

Spices

Cayenne**	Coriander	Mustard (dried)*
Chilli pepper	Cumin	Nutmeg**
Cinnamon	Fenugreek	Saffron*
Cloves**	Ginger	Turmeric

Occasionally (once per week)
**Rarely (once per month)*

Condiments

Dulse flakes	Sea salt
Kelp powder	Tempeh
Miso*	Vegetable salt
Pure vanilla bean*	Wheat-free tamari

Occasionally (once per week)

Herbal Teas

These teas have individual therapeutic values and are very beneficial. You may drink them as often as desired. Prepare teas with springwater or reverse-osmosis water. Measure 1 tsp. of herb tea into 235ml of boiled water, and allow it to stand 5 to 6 minutes. Never add sugar, milk, or lemon.

Alfalfa	Ginseng (instant)	Nettle
Avena sativa	Ginseng root	Parsley
Basil leaf	Ginseng (Siberian)	Peppermint
Chamomile	Goldenseal	Rose hip
Chickweed	Hawthorn	Skullcap
Corn silk	Horsetail	Slippery elm
Dandelion leaves	Japanese green tea	Strawberry
Dill seed	Juniper	Uva-ursi
Fenugreek	Linden	White birch
Fern	Marshmallow	White tea
Ginger	Mistletoe	

Morning Routine

Upon rising, squeeze ¼ fresh lemon into 90ml of warm to cool water.

Type-Ab Energy Drink

1 Tbsp. soy or rice protein powder
1 tsp. psyllium powder
1 tsp. stractan

Mix ingredients in 175 to 235ml of water, diluted grapefruit juice, or soy (or rice) milk. Drink one to three times daily.

Type-Ao Diet Sheet

Meat

The numbering of the columns indicates the importance of specific meats in the Type Ao diet. Number 1 is eaten most often, and number 4 is eaten less often. Meat may be baked or grilled.

1	2	2.5	3	4
Ostrich Turkey	Chicken	Lamb	Buffalo	Beef

Fish

Numbering is based on toxicity according to blood type. Number 1 is the least toxic, and 5 is the most toxic. Farm-raised fish is not desirable; wild is preferred. Fish may be baked, grilled, or boiled (do not fry).

1	1.5	2	3	4	5
Salmon	Arctic char Cod (Dec.–Apr.) Haddock Orange roughy	Grouper Kingfish Scrod Skate Trout Turbot Whitefish	Flounder Halibut Mahimahi Sole	Hake Red snapper Sturgeon Tilapia	Bass

Type Ao's should consume a total of 6 to 8 servings per week of meat and fish.

Eggs

Type Ao's can consume two eggs per week with vegetables or occasionally tofu. Free-range eggs are preferable. Whole eggs or egg whites may be poached, scrambled, or boiled; do not fry. Do not use store-bought egg whites.

Cereals

Amaranth
Brown rice cereal
Kamut
Puffed rice

Quinoa
Rice bran
Spelt
Sprouted grain cereal

Milk for Cereals
(Unsweetened)

Rice milk*
Soy milk

* *Occasionally (once per week)*

Bread and Crackers

Almond
Essene
Ezekiel (without yeast)
Kamut
Quinoa

Rice
Rice cakes
Spelt*
Sprouted wheat
Soy

* *Occasionally (once per week)*

Pasta	*or*	**Grains**
Artichoke*		Amaranth
Rice		Barley
Soy*		Basmati rice
Spelt*		Brown rice
		Buckwheat (kasha)*
		Bulgur
		Millet
		Quinoa
		Spelt*
		Teff
		Wild rice

* Occasionally (once per week)

Starchy Vegetables

Jerusalem artichokes
Potatoes (white, blue, and red)
Sweet potatoes

Dried Peas, Beans, and Lentils
(Legume Family)

Adzuki**
Cannellini*
Chickpeas**
Fava*

* Occasionally (once per week)
** Rarely (once per month)

Vegetables
(Fresh or Frozen)

Artichokes
Asparagus
Bamboo shoots
Beetroot leaves
Beetroot (small)
Belgian endive
Broccoli
(with lemon)
Brussels sprouts*
Capers*
Carrots (boiled
or raw*)
Cauliflower**
Celery
Celery root
Chicory
Chinese cabbage
Collards**
Courgettes
Cucumbers*
Daikon
Dandelion greens

Dill
Endive
Fiddleheads
Garlic clove
Green onion
Jerusalem
artichoke (fresh)
Jicama
Kale
Kohlrabi
Leeks
Lettuce (all types)
Mangetout
Mushrooms*
Okra
Olives (green)
Onions
Parsley
Peas
Peppers (green,
red, or hot*)
Radishes*

Rapini
Rocket
Savoy cabbage*
Seaweed (all types)
Shallots
Shiitake
mushrooms
Soy beans (fresh)*
Spinach (raw)
Spring onions
Sprouts (all types)
Squash (winter or
summer)
String beans
(green or yellow)
Swiss chard
Tomato
Water chestnuts
Watercress

* Occasionally (once per week)
** Rarely (once per month)

Nuts and Seeds

All varieties should be raw, unsalted, and in the shells, if possible; be sure to chew well. (A handful is about 4 Tbsp., or 60g.)

Almonds
Brazil nuts
Chestnuts*
Flaxseeds
Hazelnuts
Pecans

Pine nuts
Pumpkin seeds
Sesame seeds*
Sunflower seeds
Walnuts

Occasionally (once per week)

Nut and Seed Butters

All varieties should be raw, smooth, and without sugar or additives.

Almond
Macadamia*
Soy**
Sunflower*
Tahini (sesame butter)**

Occasionally (once per week)
**Rarely (once per month)*

Tofu

Tofu is a good source of vegetable protein. Type Ao's should eat three to five servings of organic tofu per week.

Fruits

(Fresh only or dried where indicated)

Acid	Subacid	Sweet	Neutral
Cranberries	Apples (1 or 2 per week)	Currants (black)	Breadfruit
Grapefruit	Apricots	Dates	Star apples
Lemons	Blackberries	Kumquats	Watermelon
Limes	Blueberries	Persimmons	
Pineapples	Figs (fresh)	Pomegranates	
Pomegranates	Gooseberries	Raisins (red)	
Raspberries	Grapes (blue)		
Strawberries	Kiwi		
	Loganberries		
	Mangoes		
	Nectarines		
	Papayas		
	Peaches		
	Pears		
	Plums (dark)		

Lemons may be eaten as often as you desire and may be combined with any food. Strawberries should always be eaten alone. Type Ao's should have 2 to 5 servings of fruit per day.

Juices

Juice should be freshly squeezed and kept in glass jars, or bought frozen and unsweetened. Type Ao's can have 480ml to 1.2L per day; each serving should contain ¼ juice and ¾ springwater.

Apple**	Cherry	Nectarine
Apricot	Cranberry	Papaya
Black cherry	Grape	Pineapple
Blueberry	Grapefruit	Tomato**
Celery	Lemon and water	

** *Rarely (once per month)*

Saturated and Unsaturated Fats

All oils should be cold-pressed, preferably organic, and contain no genetically modified ingredients. Don't use olive oil for cooking, as when the oil is heated, its molecular composition changes. It loses its full nutritional value and can even be carcinogenic. Grape-seed oil has a higher tolerance to heat and should be used instead.

Flaxseed oil	Safflower oil*
Grape-seed oil	Sesame oil*
Olive oil	Soy oil**
Peanut oil**	Sunflower oil*

* Occasionally (once per week)
** Rarely (once per month)

Herbs

Basil	Fennel	Sage
Bay leaf	Garlic clove	Savory
Celery seed	Lemongrass	Spring onions
Chervil	Mint	Tarragon
Chives	Oregano	Thyme
Coriander	Parsley	
Dill	Rosemary	

Spices

Anise	Coriander	Mustard seed*
Cayenne*	Cumin	Nutmeg*
Chilli pepper*	Fenugreek	Saffron*
Cinnamon	Ginger	Turmeric
Cloves*	Mustard (dried)*	

* Occasionally (once per week)

Condiments

Dulse flakes
Kelp powder
Miso**
Pure vanilla bean*
Sea salt

Tempeh**
Unprocessed apple-cider vinegar
Vegetable salt
Wheat-free tamari

* *Occasionally (once per week)*
** *Rarely (once per month)*

Herbal Teas

These teas have individual therapeutic values and are very beneficial. You may drink them as often as desired. Prepare teas with springwater or reverse-osmosis water. Measure 1 tsp. of herb tea into 235ml of boiled water, and allow it to stand 5 to 6 minutes. Never add sugar, milk, or lemon.

Alfalfa
Avena sativa
Barley
Basil leaf
Chamomile
Chickweed
Corn silk
Dandelion leaves
Fenugreek
Fern
Fig
Ginger

Ginseng (instant)
Ginseng root
Ginseng (Siberian)
Goldenseal
Hawthorn
Horsetail
Japanese green tea
Juniper
Liquorice root
Linden
Marshmallow
Mistletoe

Nettle
Parsley
Peppermint
Raspberry
Rose hip
Saint-John's-wort
Skullcap
Slippery elm
Strawberry
Uva-ursi
White birch
White tea

Morning Routine

Upon rising, squeeze ¼ fresh lemon into 90ml of cool water.

Type-Ao Energy Drink

1 Tbsp. soy or whey protein powder
1 tsp. psyllium powder
1 tsp. stractan

Mix ingredients in 175 to 235ml of water, diluted grapefruit juice, or soy (or rice) milk. Drink one to three times daily, depending on your physical energy.

Type-B Diet Sheet

Meat

The numbering of the columns indicates the importance of specific meats in the Type B diet. Number 1 is eaten most often, number 3 is eaten less often, and 5 is rarely eaten. Meat may be baked or grilled.

1	1.5	2	3	5
Lamb Ostrich Turkey	Buffalo	Calf's liver* Duck	Beef Veal Venison	Chicken

* Health-food-store purchase only

Fish

Numbering is based on toxicity according to blood type. Number 1 is the least toxic, and 4 is the most toxic. Farm-raised fish is not desirable; wild is preferred. Fish may be baked, grilled, or boiled (do not fry).

1	1.5	2	2.5	3	4
Salmon	Arctic char Cod (Dec.–Apr.) Haddock Orange roughy	Grouper Kingfish Mahimahi Scrod Skate Trout Turbot	Whitefish	Bass Flounder Halibut Sole	Hake Mackerel Red snapper Sturgeon Tilapia

Type B's should have a total of 7 to 9 servings per week of meat and fish.

Eggs

Type B's can eat four whole eggs per week with vegetables. Free-range eggs are preferred. Do not fry.

143

Cheese

Look for cheeses that don't contain food coloring, additives, or preservatives. Type B's should consume 170 to 225g per week.

Brie
Farmer cheese
Goat
Mozzarella
Ricotta

Milk Products
(150ml per week)

Goat's milk
Yogurt, plain (whole milk or 2 percent)

Cereals

Amaranth	Puffed rice
Brown rice cereal	Quinoa
Grape-Nuts	Rice bran
Kamut	Spelt
Millet	Sprouted grain cereal
Oatmeal*	

* Occasionally (once per week)

Milk for Cereals
(Unsweetened)

Almond milk
Rice milk
Soy milk*

* Occasionally (once per week)

Bread and Crackers

Essene
Ezekiel (with yeast)
Kamut
Quinoa

Rice cakes
Spelt
Sprouted wheat

Pasta   *or*   **Grains**
Artichoke
Soy
Spelt

Amaranth
Barley
Basmati rice
Brown rice
Buckwheat (kasha)*
Bulgur
Millet
Quinoa
Spelt
Teff
Wild rice

* *Occasionally (once per week)*

Starchy Vegetables

Jerusalem artichokes
Potatoes (white, blue, and red)
Sweet potatoes

Dried Peas, Beans, and Lentils
(Legume Family)

Adzuki**
Cannellini**
Chickpeas*
Fava**
Kidney**

* Occasionally (once per week)
** Rarely (once per month)

Vegetables
(Fresh or Frozen)

Artichokes
Asparagus
Bamboo shoots
Beetroot leaves
Beetroot (small)
Belgian endive
Broccoli
(with lemon)
Brussels sprouts
Cabbage (white*
or red)
Carrots (raw
or boiled)
Cauliflower**
Celery
Celery root
Chicory
Chinese cabbage
Collards
Courgettes
Cucumber
Daikon

Dandelion greens
Dill
Endive
Fiddleheads
Garlic clove
Green onion
Jerusalem
artichoke (fresh)
Jicama
Kale
Kohlrabi
Leek
Lettuce (all types)
Mangetout
Mushrooms
Okra
Olives (green)
Onions
Parsley
Peas
Peppers (green,
red, or hot*)

Radishes
Rapini
Rocket
Savoy cabbage
Seaweed (all types)
Shallots
Shiitake
mushrooms
Spinach (raw)
Sprouts (all types)
Squash (winter
or summer)
String beans
(green or yellow)
Swede
Swiss chard
Tomato**
Water chestnuts*
Watercress

* Occasionally (once per week)
** Rarely (once per month)

Nuts and Seeds

All varieties should be raw, unsalted, and in the shells, if possible; be sure to chew well. (A handful is about 4 Tbsp., or 60g.)

Almonds	Pine nuts
Brazil nuts	Pistachios*
Chestnuts*	Pumpkin seeds
Flaxseeds	Sunflower seeds
Hazelnuts	Walnuts
Pecans	

* *Occasionally (once per week)*

Nut and Seed Butters

All varieties should be raw, smooth, and without sugar or additives.

Almond
Macadamia
Sunflower
Tahini (sesame butter)*

* *Occasionally (once per week)*

Tofu

Tofu is a good source of vegetable protein. Type B's should eat one to two servings of organic tofu in the midmorning per week.

Fruits
(Fresh only or dried where indicated)

Acid	Subacid	Sweet	Neutral
Cranberries	Apples*	Currants (black)	Breadfruit
Grapefruit	Apricots	Dates	Star apples
Lemons	Blackberries	Figs (dried)	Watermelon
Limes	Blueberries	Kumquats	
Pineapples	Cherries	Persimmons	
Pomegranates	Figs (fresh)	Pomegranates	
Raspberries	Gooseberries	Raisins (red)	
Strawberries	Grapes (blue)		
	Kiwi		
	Loganberries		
	Mangoes		
	Nectarines		
	Papayas		
	Peaches		
	Pears		
	Plums (dark)		

Occasionally (once per week)

Lemons may be eaten as often as you desire and may be combined with any food. Strawberries should always be eaten alone.

Juices

Juice should be freshly squeezed and kept in glass jars, or bought frozen and unsweetened. Type B's can have 480ml to 1.65L per day; each serving should contain ¼ juice and ¾ springwater.

Apricot	Cherry	Papaya
Black cherry	Cranberry	Peach
Blueberry	Grape	Pineapple
Carrot	Grapefruit	
Celery	Lemon and water	

Saturated and Unsaturated Fats

All oils should be cold-pressed, preferably organic, and contain no genetically modified ingredients. Don't use olive oil for cooking, as when the oil is heated, its molecular composition changes. It loses its full nutritional value and can even be carcinogenic. Grape-seed oil has a higher tolerance to heat and should be used instead.

Flaxseed oil	Sesame oil*
Grape-seed oil	Soy oil*
Olive oil	Sunflower oil*
Safflower oil*	

* Occasionally (once per week)

The D'Adamo Institute created a healthy spread (the Institute's Spread) that can be used in place of margarine or pure butter. Type B's should use ¼ to ½ teaspoon three times per week.

Institute's Spread

110g sweet butter
60ml grape-seed or olive oil
1 vitamin E capsule
1 lecithin capsule

Whip ingredients together and refrigerate.

Herbs

Basil	Fennel	Rosemary
Bay leaf	Garlic clove	Sage
Celery seed	Lemongrass	Savory
Chervil	Marjoram	Spring onions
Chives	Mint	Tarragon
Coriander	Oregano	Thyme
Dill	Parsley	

Spices

Anise	Cumin	Paprika*
Cayenne*	Curry powder*	Pepper*
Chilli pepper	Fenugreek	Saffron
Cinnamon	Ginger	Turmeric
Cloves	Mustard (dried)	
Coriander	Nutmeg*	

Occasionally (once per week)

Condiments

Dulse flakes	Unprocessed apple-cider vinegar*
Kelp powder	Vegetable salt
Miso**	Wheat-free tamari
Pure vanilla bean*	
Sea salt	

Occasionally (once per week)
**Rarely (once per month)*

Herbal Teas

These teas have individual therapeutic values and are very beneficial. You may drink them as often as desired. Prepare teas with springwater or reverse-osmosis water. Measure 1 tsp. of herb tea into 235ml of boiled water, and allow it to stand 5 to 6 minutes. Never add sugar, milk, or lemon.

Alfalfa	Ginseng (Siberian)	Nettle
Avena sativa	Goldenseal	Parsley
Basil leaf	Hawthorn	Peppermint
Chamomile	Holy thistle	Rockrose
Chickweed	Horsetail	Rose hip
Corn silk	Japanese green tea	Skullcap
Dandelion leaves	Juniper	Slippery elm
Dill seed	Lady's mantle	Solomon's seal
Fenugreek	Liquorice root	Strawberry
Fern	Linden	Tanacetum
Ginger	Marshmallow	Uva-ursi
Ginseng (instant)	Maté	White birch
Ginseng root	Mistletoe	White tea

Morning Routine

Upon rising, squeeze ¼ fresh lemon into 100ml of cool water.

Type-B Energy Drink

1 Tbsp. soy, whey, or rice protein powder
1 tsp. psyllium powder
1 tsp. stractan
1 tsp. flaxseed oil

Mix ingredients in 175 to 235ml of water, diluted grapefruit juice, or soy (or rice) milk. Drink one to three times daily.

Type-Ba Diet Sheet

Meat

The numbering of the columns indicates the importance of specific meats in the Type Ba diet. Number 1 is eaten most often, and number 4 is eaten less often. Meat may be baked or grilled.

1	2	2.5	3	4
Ostrich Turkey	Buffalo	Lamb	Beef	Chicken

Fish

Numbering is based on toxicity according to blood type. Number 1 is the least toxic, and 5 is the most toxic. Farm-raised fish is not desirable; wild is preferred. Fish may be baked, grilled, or boiled (do not fry).

1	1.5	2	3	4	5
Salmon	Arctic char Cod (Dec.–Apr.) Haddock Orange roughy	Grouper Kingfish Scrod Skate Trout Turbot	Bass Halibut Mahimahi Skate Sole	Hake Red snapper Sturgeon Tilapia	Mackerel

Eggs

Type Ba's can eat three eggs per week with tofu or vegetables. Use egg whites only (don't use store-bought egg whites). Free-range eggs are preferred. Eggs may be poached, scrambled, or hard-boiled. Do not fry.

Starch

Avoid products that contain wheat.

Cereals

Amaranth	Quinoa
Brown rice cereal	Rice bran
Kamut	Spelt
Puffed rice	Sprouted grain cereal

Milk for Cereals
(Unsweetened)

Almond milk*
Rice milk
Soy milk

* *Occasionally (once per week)*

Bread and Crackers
(Yeast Free)

Essene	Soy
Ezekiel (without yeast)	Spelt*
Kamut	Sprouted wheat
Quinoa	

* *Occasionally (once per week)*

Pasta	*or*	**Grains**
Artichoke		Amaranth
Rice		Barley
Soy		Basmati rice
Spelt		Brown rice
		Buckwheat (kasha)*
		Bulgur
		Millet
		Quinoa
		Spelt
		Teff
		Wild rice

* Occasionally (once per week)

Starchy Vegetables

Jerusalem artichokes
Potatoes (white, blue, and red)
Sweet potatoes

Dried Peas, Beans, and Lentils
(Legume Family)

Adzuki*
Cannellini*
Chickpeas*
Fava*

* Occasionally (once per week)

Vegetables
(Fresh or Frozen)

Artichokes
Asparagus
Bamboo shoots
Beetroot leaves
Beetroot (small)
Belgian endive
Broccoli
(with lemon)
Brussels sprouts*
Capers
Carrots (raw
or boiled)
Celery
Celery root
Chicory
Chinese cabbage
Collards*
Courgettes
Cucumber
Daikon
Dandelion greens

Dill
Endive
Fiddleheads
Garlic clove
Green onion
Jerusalem
artichoke (fresh)
Jicama
Kale
Kohlrabi
Leeks
Lettuce (all types)
Mangetout
Okra
Olives (green)
Onions
Parsley
Peas
Peppers (green,
red, or hot**)
Radishes*

Rapini
Rocket
Savoy cabbage*
Seaweed (all types)
Shallots
Shiitake
mushrooms
Spinach (raw)
Spring onions
Sprouts (all types)
Squash (winter
or summer)
String beans
(green or yellow)
Swede
Swiss chard
Tomato**
Water chestnuts
Watercress

* *Occasionally (once per week)*
** *Rarely (once per month)*

For a wonderful vegetable soup, try the Vegetarian Soup recipe in Chapter 11. Type Ba's can eat this soup one to seven times per week.

Nuts and Seeds

All varieties should be raw, unsalted, and in the shells, if possible; be sure to chew well. (A handful is about 4 Tbsp., or 60g.)

Almonds	Pistachios*
Chestnuts*	Pumpkin seeds
Flaxseeds	Sunflower seeds
Pecans	Walnuts
Pine nuts	

Occasionally (once per week)

Nut and Seed Butters

All varieties should be raw, smooth, and without sugar or additives.

Almond
Macadamia
Sunflower
Tahini (sesame butter)*

Occasionally (once per week)

Tofu

Tofu is a good source of vegetable protein. Type Ba's should eat two to three servings of organic tofu per week.

Fruits
(Fresh only or dried where indicated)

Acid	Subacid	Sweet	Neutral
Cranberries	Apples**	Currants (black)	Breadfruit
Grapefruit	Apricots	Dates	Star apples
Lemons	Blackberries	Figs (dried)	Watermelon
Limes	Blueberries	Kumquats	
Pineapples	Cherries	Persimmons	
Pomegranates	Figs (fresh)	Pomegranates	
Raspberries	Gooseberries	Raisins (red)	
Strawberries	Grapes (blue)		
	Kiwi		
	Loganberries		
	Mangoes		
	Nectarines		
	Papayas		
	Peaches		
	Pears		
	Plums (dark)		

** *Rarely (once per month)*

Lemons may be eaten as often as you desire and may be combined with any food. Strawberries should always be eaten alone.

Juices

Juice should be freshly squeezed and kept in glass jars, or bought frozen and unsweetened. Type Ba's can have 480ml to 1.65L per day; each serving should contain ¼ juice and ¾ springwater.

Apricot	Cherry	Lemon and water
Black cherry	Cranberry	Papaya
Blueberry	Grape	Pineapple
Celery	Grapefruit	

Saturated and Unsaturated Fats

All oils should be cold-pressed, preferably organic, and contain no genetically modified ingredients. Don't use olive oil for cooking, as when the oil is heated, its molecular composition changes. It loses its full nutritional value and can even be carcinogenic. Grape-seed oil has a higher tolerance to heat and should be used instead.

Flaxseed oil	Sesame oil*
Grape-seed oil	Soy oil*
Olive oil	Sunflower oil*
Safflower oil*	

* Occasionally (once per week)

The D'Adamo Institute created a healthy spread (the Institute's Spread) that can be used in place of margarine or pure butter. Type Ba's should use ⅛ teaspoon two times per week.

Institute's Spread

110g sweet butter
60ml grape-seed or olive oil
1 vitamin E capsule
1 lecithin capsule

Whip ingredients together and refrigerate.

Herbs

Basil	Fennel	Sage
Bay leaf	Garlic clove	Savory
Celery seed	Lemongrass	Spring onions
Chervil	Mint	Tarragon
Chives	Oregano	Thyme
Coriander	Parsley	
Dill	Rosemary	

Spices

Anise	Coriander	Ginger
Chilli pepper**	Cumin	Mustard (dried)*
Cinnamon	Curry powder**	Saffron*
Cloves*	Fenugreek	Turmeric

* Occasionally (once per week)
** Rarely (once per month)

Condiments

Dulse flakes	Sea salt
Kelp powder	Tempeh*
Miso*	Vegetable salt
Pure vanilla bean*	Wheat-free tamari

* Occasionally (once per week)

Herbal Teas

These teas have individual therapeutic values and are very beneficial. You may drink them as often as desired. Prepare teas with springwater or reverse-osmosis water. Measure 1 tsp. of herb tea into 235ml of boiled water, and allow it to stand 5 to 6 minutes. Never add sugar, milk, or lemon.

Alfalfa	Ginseng (Siberian)	Nettle
Avena sativa	Goldenseal	Parsley
Chamomile	Hawthorn	Peppermint
Chickweed	Holy thistle	Rose hip*
Dandelion leaves	Horsetail	Skullcap
Fenugreek	Japanese green tea	Slippery elm
Fern	Liquorice root	Strawberry
Ginger	Linden	Uva-ursi
Ginseng (instant)	Marshmallow	White tea
Ginseng root	Maté	

* Occasionally (once per week)

Morning Routine

Upon rising, squeeze ¼ fresh lemon into 100ml of warm to cool water.

Type-Ba Energy Drink

1 Tbsp. soy or rice protein powder
1 tsp. psyllium powder
1 tsp. stractan

Mix ingredients in 175 to 235ml of water, diluted grapefruit juice, or soy (or rice) milk. Drink one to three times daily.

Type-Bo Diet Sheet

Meat

The numbering of the columns indicates the importance of specific meats in the Type Bo diet. Number 1 is eaten most often, and number 4 is eaten less often. Meat may be baked or grilled.

1	1.5	2	2.5	3	4
Heart (beef or lamb) Lamb Ostrich Turkey	Buffalo	Beef Duck Veal	Calf's liver* Venison	Rabbit	Chicken

* Health-food-store purchase only

Fish

Numbering is based on toxicity according to blood type. Number 1 is the least toxic, and 4 is the most toxic. Farm-raised fish is not desirable; wild is preferred. Fish may be baked, grilled, or boiled (do not fry).

1	1.5	2	2.5	3	4
Salmon	Arctic char Cod (Dec.–Apr.) Haddock Orange roughy	Grouper Kingfish Mahimahi Scrod Skate Trout Turbot	Halibut Sardines* Sturgeon Whitefish	Flounder Mackerel Shad Sole	Hake Red snapper Tilapia

* In water

Type Bo's should have a total of 8 to 10 servings per week of meat and fish.

Eggs

Type Bo's can eat four whole eggs per week with vegetables. Free-range eggs are preferred. Do not fry.

Cheese

Look for cheeses that don't contain food coloring, additives, or preservatives. Type Bo's can have 5 to 6 oz. per week.

Goat**
Mozzarella*
Ricotta*

Occasionally (once per week)
*** Rarely (once per month)*

Milk Products
(3 oz. per week)

Goat's milk
Yogurt, plain (whole milk or 2 percent)

Cereals

Amaranth	Puffed rice
Brown rice cereal	Quinoa
Grape-Nuts	Rice bran
Kamut	Spelt
Millet	Sprouted grain cereal
Oatmeal*	

Occasionally (once per week)

Milk for Cereals
(Unsweetened)

Almond milk
Rice milk
Soy milk**

** *Rarely (once per month)*

Bread and Crackers

Almond	Rice
Essene	Rice cakes
Ezekiel (without yeast)	Spelt
Quinoa	Sprouted wheat

Pasta	*or*	**Grains**
Artichoke		Amaranth
Rice		Barley
Soy**		Basmati rice
Spelt		Brown rice
		Bulgur
		Millet
		Quinoa
		Spelt
		Teff
		Wild rice

** *Rarely (once per month)*

Starchy Vegetables

Jerusalem artichokes
Potatoes (white, blue, and red)
Sweet potatoes

Dried Peas, Beans, and Lentils
(Legume Family)

Cannellini**
Chickpeas**
Fava**
Kidney**
Lentil**

** *Rarely (once per month)*

Vegetables
(Fresh or Frozen)

Artichokes
Asparagus
Bamboo shoots
Beetroot leaves
Beetroot (small)
Belgian endive
Broccoli
(with lemon)
Brussels sprouts*
Cabbage (white**)
Capers
Carrots (raw
or boiled)
Cauliflower**
Celery
Celery root
Chicory
Chinese cabbage
Collards
Courgettes
Cucumber
Daikon

Dandelion greens
Dill
Endive
Fiddleheads
Garlic clove
Green onion
Jerusalem
artichoke (fresh)
Jicama
Kale
Kohlrabi
Leeks
Lettuce (all types)
Mangetout
Mushrooms*
Okra
Olives (green)
Onions
Parsley
Peas
Peppers (green,
red, or hot)

Radishes
Rapini
Rocket
Savoy cabbage**
Seaweed (all types)
Shallots
Shiitake
mushrooms
Spinach (raw)
Spring onions
Sprouts (all types)
Squash (winter
or summer)
String beans (green
or yellow)
Swede
Swiss chard
Tomato**
Water chestnuts
Watercress

* *Occasionally (once per week)*
** *Rarely (once per month)*

For a wonderful vegetable soup, try the Vegetarian Soup recipe in Chapter 11. Type Bo's can eat this soup one to seven times per week.

Nuts and Seeds

All varieties should be raw, unsalted, and in the shells, if possible; be sure to chew well. (A handful is about 4 Tbsp., or 60g.)

Almonds	Pine nuts
Brazil nuts	Pistachios*
Chestnuts*	Pumpkin seeds
Flaxseeds	Sesame seeds**
Hazelnuts	Sunflower seeds
Pecans	Walnuts

* Occasionally (once per week)
** Rarely (once per month)

Nut and Seed Butters

All varieties should be raw, smooth, and without sugar or additives.

Almond
Macadamia
Sunflower
Tahini (sesame butter)**

** Rarely (once per month)

Tofu

Tofu is a good source of vegetable protein. Type Bo's should eat one to two servings of organic tofu per week.

Fruits

(Fresh only or dried where indicated)

Acid	Subacid	Sweet	Neutral
Cranberries	Apples (1 or 2 per week)	Currants (black)	Breadfruit
Grapefruit	Apricots	Dates	Star apples
Lemons	Blackberries	Figs (dried)	Watermelon
Limes	Blueberries	Kumquats	
Pineapples	Cherries	Persimmons	
Pomegranates	Figs (fresh)	Pomegranates	
Raspberries	Gooseberries	Raisins (red)	
Strawberries	Grapes (blue)		
	Kiwi		
	Mangoes		
	Nectarines		
	Papayas		
	Peaches		
	Pears		
	Plums (dark)		

Lemons may be eaten as often as you desire and may be combined with any food. Strawberries should always be eaten alone.

Juices

Juice should be freshly squeezed and kept in glass jars, or bought frozen and unsweetened. Each serving should contain ¼ juice and ¾ springwater.

Apricot	Cherry	Nectarine
Black cherry	Cranberry	Peach
Blueberry	Grape	Pineapple
Carrot	Grapefruit	
Celery	Lemon and water	

Saturated and Unsaturated Fats

All oils should be cold-pressed, preferably organic, and contain no genetically modified ingredients. Don't use olive oil for cooking, as when the oil is heated, its molecular composition changes. It loses its full nutritional value and can even be carcinogenic. Grape-seed oil has a higher tolerance to heat and should be used instead.

Flaxseed oil	Safflower oil*
Grape-seed oil	Sesame oil*
Olive oil	Sunflower oil*

* Occasionally (once per week)

The D'Adamo Institute created a healthy spread (the Institute's Spread) that can be used in place of margarine or pure butter. Type Bo's should use ½ teaspoon three to four times per week.

Institute's Spread

110g sweet butter
60ml grape-seed or olive oil
1 vitamin E capsule
1 lecithin capsule

Whip ingredients together and refrigerate.

Herbs

Basil	Fennel	Rosemary
Bay leaf	Garlic clove	Sage
Celery seed	Lemongrass	Savory
Chervil	Marjoram	Spring onions
Chives	Mint	Tarragon
Coriander	Oregano	Thyme
Dill	Parsley	

Spices

Anise	Coriander	Mustard (dried)
Cayenne*	Cumin	Nutmeg
Chilli pepper*	Curry powder*	Paprika*
Cinnamon	Fenugreek	Saffron*
Cloves	Ginger	Turmeric

* Occasionally (once per week)

Condiments

Dulse flakes	Vegetable salt
Kelp powder	Wheat-free tamari
Sea salt	
Unprocessed apple-cider vinegar*	

* Occasionally (once per week)

Herbal Teas

These teas have individual therapeutic values and are very beneficial. You may drink them as often as desired. Prepare teas with springwater or reverse-osmosis water. Measure 1 tsp. of herb tea into 235ml of boiled water, and allow it to stand 5 to 6 minutes. Never add sugar, milk, or lemon.

Alfalfa	Ginseng root	Nettle
Avena sativa	Goldenseal	Parsley
Basil leaf	Hawthorn	Peppermint
Chamomile	Holy thistle	Rose hip*
Chickweed	Horsetail	Skullcap
Corn silk	Japanese green tea	Slippery elm
Dandelion leaves	Juniper	Solomon's seal
Dill seed	Liquorice root	Strawberry
Fenugreek	Linden	Tanacetum
Fern	Marshmallow	Uva-ursi
Ginger	Maté	White birch
Ginseng (instant)	Mistletoe	White tea

* Occasionally (once per week)

Morning Routine

Upon rising, squeeze ½ fresh lemon into 3½ oz. of cool to cold water.

Type-Bo Energy Drink

1 Tbsp. whey protein powder
1 tsp. psyllium powder
1 tsp. stractan

Mix ingredients in 175 to 235ml of water, diluted grapefruit juice, or soy (or rice) milk. Drink two to three times daily.

Type-AB Diet Sheet

Meat

The numbering of the columns indicates the importance of specific meats in the Type AB diet. Number 1 is eaten most often, and number 3 is eaten less often. Meat may be baked or grilled.

1	2	2.5	3
Ostrich Turkey	Buffalo Duck Venison	Calf's liver* Lamb	Beef Chicken

* Health-food-store purchase only

Fish

Numbering is based on toxicity according to blood type. Number 1 is the least toxic, and 4 is the most toxic. Farm-raised fish is not desirable; wild is preferred. Fish may be baked, grilled, or boiled (do not fry).

1	1.5	2	2.5	3	4
Salmon	Arctic char Haddock Orange roughy	Grouper Kingfish Scrod Skate Trout Turbot	Whitefish	Bass Flounder Halibut Sole	Hake Mackerel Red snapper Sturgeon Tilapia

Type AB's should consume a total of 5 to 7 servings per week of meat and fish.

Eggs

Type AB's can eat three to four whole eggs per week with vegetables or tofu. Free-range eggs are preferred. Do not fry.

Cheese

Look for cheeses that don't contain food coloring, additives, or preservatives.

Feta**
Mozzarella**
Ricotta**

** *Rarely (once per month)*

Cereals

Amaranth
Brown rice cereal
Kamut
Millet
Oatmeal**

Puffed rice
Quinoa
Rice bran
Spelt
Sprouted grain cereal

** *Rarely (once per month)*

Milk for Cereals
(Unsweetened)

Almond milk
Rice milk
Soy milk

Bread and Crackers
(Yeast Free)

Essene
Ezekiel
Kamut
Quinoa

Rice cakes
Spelt
Soy

Pasta	*or*	**Grains**
Rice		Amaranth
Soy		Barley
Spelt		Basmati rice
		Brown rice
		Buckwheat (kasha)
		Bulgur
		Millet
		Quinoa
		Spelt
		Teff
		Wild rice

Starchy Vegetables

Jerusalem artichokes
Potatoes (white, blue, and red)
Sweet potatoes

Dried Peas, Beans, and Lentils
(Legume Family)

Adzuki*	Kidney*
Cannellini*	Lentil**
Chickpeas*	Peanut
Fava*	Soy*

* Occasionally (once per week)
** Rarely (once per month)

Vegetables
(Fresh or Frozen)

Artichokes
Asparagus
Bamboo shoots
Beetroot leaves
Beetroot (small)
Belgian endive
Broccoli (with lemon)
Brussels sprouts
Capers*
Carrots (raw* or boiled)
Cauliflower*
Celery
Celery root
Chicory
Chinese cabbage
Collards
Courgettes
Cucumbers*
Daikon

Dandelion greens
Dill
Endive
Fiddleheads
Garlic clove
Green onion
Jerusalem artichoke (fresh)
Jicama
Kale
Kohlrabi
Leeks
Lettuce (all types)
Mangetout
Mushrooms*
Okra
Olives (green)
Onions
Parsley
Peas
Peppers (green, red,

or hot*)
Radishes
Rapini
Rocket
Savoy cabbage*
Seaweed (all types)
Shallots
Shiitake mushrooms
Soy beans (fresh)
Spring onions
Spinach (raw)
Sprouts (all types)
Squash (winter or summer)
String beans (green or yellow)
Swiss chard
Tomato*
Water chestnuts*
Watercress

Occasionally (once per week)

Nuts and Seeds

All varieties should be raw, unsalted, and in the shells, if possible; be sure to chew well. (A handful is about 4 Tbsp., or 60g.)

Almonds
Brazil nuts
Chestnuts*
Flaxseeds

Hazelnuts
Pecans
Pine nuts
Pistachios*

Pumpkin seeds
Sesame seeds*
Sunflower seeds
Walnuts

Occasionally (once per week)

Nut and Seed Butters

All varieties should be raw, smooth, and without sugar or additives.

Almond
Macadamia
Soy
Sunflower*
Tahini (sesame butter)*

Occasionally (once per week)

Fruits
(Fresh only or dried where indicated)

Acid	Subacid	Sweet	Neutral
Cranberries	Apricots	Currants (black)	Breadfruit
Grapefruit	Blackberries	Dates	Star apples
Lemons	Blueberries	Figs (dried)	Watermelon
Limes	Cherries	Kumquats	
Pineapples	Figs (fresh)	Raisins (red)	
Pomegranates	Gooseberries		
Raspberries	Grapes (blue)		
Strawberries	Guava		
	Kiwi		
	Loganberries		
	Mangoes		
	Nectarines		
	Papayas		
	Peaches		
	Pears		
	Plums (dark)		

Lemons may be eaten as often as you desire and may be combined with any food. Strawberries should always be eaten alone.

Juices

Juice should be freshly squeezed and kept in glass jars, or bought frozen and unsweetened. Type AB's can have 480ml to 1.65L per day total; each serving should contain ¼ juice and ¾ springwater.

Apricot	Celery	Lemon and water
Black cherry	Cranberry	Papaya
Blueberry	Grape	Pineapple
Carrot	Grapefruit	

Saturated and Unsaturated Fats

All oils should be cold-pressed, preferably organic, and contain no genetically modified ingredients. Don't use olive oil for cooking, as when the oil is heated, its molecular composition changes. It loses its full nutritional value and can even be carcinogenic. Grape-seed oil has a higher tolerance to heat and should be used instead.

Flaxseed oil	Sesame oil*
Grape-seed oil	Soy oil*
Olive oil	Sunflower oil*
Safflower oil*	

* Occasionally (once per week)

Herbs

Basil	Fennel	Rosemary
Bay leaf	Garlic clove	Sage
Celery seed	Lemongrass	Savory
Chervil	Marjoram	Spring onions
Chives	Mint	Tarragon
Coriander	Oregano	Thyme
Dill	Parsley	

Spices

Anise	Cumin	Nutmeg*
Cayenne*	Curry powder*	Paprika*
Chilli pepper*	Fenugreek	Saffron*
Cinnamon	Ginger	Turmeric
Cloves	Horseradish*	
Coriander	Mustard (dried)	

* Occasionally (once per week)

Condiments

Dulse flakes	Sea salt
Kelp powder	Tempeh*
Miso*	Vegetable salt
Pure vanilla bean*	Wheat-free tamari

* Occasionally (once per week)

Herbal Teas

These teas have individual therapeutic values and are very beneficial. You may drink them as often as desired. Prepare teas with springwater or reverse-osmosis water. Measure 1 tsp. of herb tea into 235ml of boiled water, and allow it to stand 5 to 6 minutes. Never add sugar, milk, or lemon.

Alfalfa	Ginseng root	Parsley
Avena sativa	Goldenseal	Peppermint
Barley	Hawthorn	Rose hip
Basil leaf	Holy thistle	Saint-John's-wort
Burdock	Horsetail	Skullcap
Chamomile	Japanese green tea	Slippery elm
Chickweed	Juniper	Strawberry
Corn silk	Lady's mantle	Uva-ursi
Daisy	Liquorice root	White birch
Dandelion leaves	Linden	White tea
Dill seed	Marshmallow	Wormwood
Fenugreek	Maté	Yellow dock
Fern	Mistletoe	
Ginger	Nettle	

Morning Routine

Upon rising, squeeze ¼ fresh lemon into 90ml of cool water.

Type-AB Energy Drink

1 Tbsp. soy or rice protein powder
1 tsp. psyllium powder
1 tsp. stractan

Mix ingredients in 175 to 235ml of water, diluted grapefruit juice, or soy (or rice) milk. Drink one to three times daily if you feel fatigued or are overweight or constipated.

CHAPTER NINE

How to Create Your Prevention Program

Few people can plunge straight into a new menu pattern. The changes are too vast and demanding, and they are likely to give up after struggling for a few days or weeks. In this chapter, I'll guide you as you modify your diet and lifestyle. The key is to go slowly, allowing your body and mind time to adjust. In most cases, it will take about a year to comfortably move into your new regimen, regardless of your blood type. (Please note: This program may vary, depending upon a person's current state of health.)

Type O

Level 1

Eliminate processed and refined foods. Substitute Kamut, quinoa, spelt, and Ezekiel breads for breads made of white or enriched flour; and do not eat processed cereals. Introduce sprouted wheat and rice cereals, such as millet or oatmeal, to replace sugared and puffed breakfast cereals.

Reduce beef and pork products. Select animal protein from buffalo, lamb, calf's liver, chicken, turkey, the internal organs of organically raised cattle (kidney, heart, and lungs), and fish. Eliminate commercially produced dairy products, and choose almond and rice milk instead of cow's milk.

Eliminate fried foods. Reduce alcohol consumption and cigarette smoking. Substitute honey for white or brown sugar.

Evaluate your exercise program. Your goal is to create a vigorous regimen appropriate to your age and physical condition. An hour (depending on your condition) of exercise such as jogging, swimming, bicycling, or gymnastics every day will greatly benefit you now. Work into this step over a period of a month to a month and a half.

Level 2

Animal protein should be eaten once or twice a day. Choose from the recommended selection in level 5. Soft cheeses (including ricotta, farmer, cottage, and mozzarella) may now be eaten five times a week, but start to slowly reduce your usual intake by eliminating it every other day. A half glass of rice or almond milk may be drunk every day, and you can also have six eggs a week and yogurt twice weekly. In addition, you may eat sprouted-wheat products as often as you like, and you can choose from such cereals as millet, oatmeal, and bran.

If you are younger than 30, you may use butter made from raw cream, but do so in moderation. Type O's over 30 (the age at which your body's systems begin to become more susceptible to the buildup of fatty deposits in your circulatory system) should switch to margarines made of polyunsaturated oils such as safflower or sunflower. Cold-pressed olive oil can be mixed with lemon juice and your choice of herbs for salad dressing.

Sea salt may be used in moderation, but do not use kelp powder because its rich iodine content may overstimulate your thyroid gland and increase your metabolic rate.

Vegetarian lunches should be introduced into your diet once or twice a week.

This step can be adapted over a period of two months. Once you've reached this stage successfully, there will be few changes as you work toward level 5, the ideal diet.

Level 3

Refer to level 2 for your allowed intake of animal protein. Cow's milk should now be reduced or entirely eliminated, choosing either almond or rice milk. You can drink several glasses of almond or rice milk a day. Soft cheeses mentioned in level 2 may be eaten three times a week; yogurt once a week. You should now lower your intake of eggs from six to four per week; if your energy level is high, consume only one to two eggs a week.

Lunches should now be vegetarian two to three times a week. Make sure you use at least a tablespoon of olive oil in your salad dressing to assist digestion and promote elimination.

To stimulate your body, take cold showers, hip baths (fill the bath with enough tepid water to cover the buttocks and hips), and saunas regularly. All increase circulation and help detoxification.

Unless you're suffering from a serious illness, you can spend three to four months working up to this level.

Level 4

Continue to follow the regimen outlined in level 3 with these changes: Lunch should be your largest meal and should now be totally vegetarian. In addition, eat a square of tofu with every meal for additional protein. You can remain at this level for three to four months.

Level 5

The ideal O diet is as follows: oatmeal, spelt, Kamut, quinoa, cornmeal, millet, or bran for breakfast with rice or almond milk and a dab of honey. Bread may be selected from spelt, Kamut, quinoa, Ezekiel, or sprouted wheat.

Lunch (or the meal other than the main meal) should be vegetarian, consisting of mixed salads and sprouts with seeds and almonds, or fish. Five eggs are your weekly allowance.

The main meal of the day should be meat. The best balance is veal once a week; calf's liver and lamb once every two weeks; and chicken, turkey, buffalo, or fish as many times as you wish. Remember, you must adapt your protein intake to your individual condition.

Type A

Level 1

This is an evaluation step for those who are not yet following a healthy dietary regimen and are still eating commercially processed foods. Most Type A's will have a long journey to level 5, with many foods to eliminate from their diets as they make the adjustment to a vegetarian lifestyle. They will have to be patient in altering their menu, but it's not impossible, nor even terribly difficult. I, myself, am an A and a product of a good Italian family, meaning that I had my share of pasta, sausages, and prosciutto to give up! Even though I had fond memories of spaghetti and clam sauce, when I decided to change my eating habits, it took only about six weeks to reeducate my taste buds and embrace a new way of eating.

Take it from me: your palate quickly loses its desire for certain tastes. It's your thoughts that you must master. Control your thoughts and in a short period of time you can switch from, for example, scungilli to a fresh mixed salad without feeling deprived.

Before you try to eliminate meat and dairy products from your diet, first substitute better-quality equivalents for the foods you're now eating. Replace white flour with spelt flour; and choose whole-grain breads and cereals, such as whole wheat, rye, rolled oats, cornmeal, millet, cracked wheat, and buckwheat. Canned foods should be replaced by fresh fruits and vegetables. Foods that have been preserved, flavored, or colored or are chemically synthesized should be totally eliminated.

Buy your own pure ingredients: bake your own cakes, prepare your own pasta dinners, or steam your own brown rice. Think about what you're putting into your body. When you're eating, be aware that food is fuel and a poor grade of fuel is going to clog and rob your human machine of its potential energy and efficiency. Try to control your cravings. Be patient, and focus on abundant health.

The same kind of discretion should apply when selecting meats. It's crucial to avoid all packed meats such as canned ham, frankfurters, and frozen fish. These foods are usually preserved with salt and chemicals such as sodium nitrite, which has been linked to cancer. When shopping, be sure to buy only grade-A meats, with no additives. Most supermarkets carry free-range meats that contain no antibiotics or other chemicals. Meat should also be well sealed: exposure to air reduces its nutritional value. If you are buying a lot of red meats, such as chopped beef, steaks, roasts, or pork products, think about switching to veal, lamb, chicken, and turkey. The latter choices are leaner and have less uric acid as well as smaller concentrations of steroids and antibiotics. Fish is also lean and a purer food.

Your main consideration in buying food should be whether it's in its purest, simplest state—a fruit should be as close to the state in which it fell from the tree, a vegetable the state it grew from the earth, and so on.

Other factors that affect your health and that should now be examined are the amount of alcohol you drink, the number of cigarettes you smoke per day, and your current exercise program. Hard alcohol, which robs the body of many nutrients and debilitates the liver, should be eliminated and replaced with moderate quantities of red or white wine. Cigarettes weaken the lungs, destroy vitamin C (which can lower your resistance to disease), and have been proven to contain cancer-causing agents. If you really want to recover your health fully, try to cut down with the goal of eventually eliminating cigarette smoking.

Lastly, evaluate your current exercise program. Do you work out? How much? Are you exerting yourself? Remember that Type A's should find peace through physical exercise and shouldn't be stressing themselves by attempting to be marathon runners or a Michael Phelps. Take up meditation and tai chi or yoga, which elongates muscles and reduces tension.

Type A's should remain at this level for one to two months.

Level 2

At this level, you'll narrow your selection of foods. Your choice of meats should now only include veal, lamb, chicken, turkey, or fish. Beef and pork products should be completely eliminated. Whole-wheat products and wheat-derived grains that were introduced in level 1 should now be alternated with soy products. For instance, spelt or Ezekiel breads may be eaten three or four times a week; on the other days, select a soy loaf. Soybeans and soy flakes or granules should be substituted for millet, cracked wheat, or buckwheat. A square of tofu should also be eaten with every meal.

In addition, the amount of dairy products you consume should be reduced: milk should be diluted with water, soft cheeses substituted for hard cheeses, eggs limited to four or five a week, and yogurt eaten only twice per week. Soy milk may be substituted for cow's milk. Items made from goat's milk are more beneficial than cow's milk, cheese, and yogurt.

You should start eating vegetables steamed, not raw. This will help your body adapt to these highly laxative foods and have a gentler effect on your bowels than raw vegetables. As your body adjusts to fresh foods, which may happen at this level or later in the program, you can eat your vegetables either steamed or raw.

Lunch should gradually become a vegetarian meal. If you aren't ready to have raw salads as your meal, make a plate of steamed vegetables. If your body readily adapts to raw foods, then prepare a salad to your liking, but omit your favorite salad dressing. From this point on, use only oil and lemon and a few herbs such as rosemary, oregano, basil, or dill. Cider vinegar especially should be avoided, as it's too acidic for your body. Sea salt should be used instead of regular table salt. Kelp powder, which is beneficial to a hyperactive thyroid, may also be used as a condiment on salads, vegetables, or meat dishes.

Remain at this level for about two months.

Level 3

All animal protein except chicken and fish should now be eliminated, and it's recommended that you reduce your intake to twice a week. The following types of fish are listed in order of preference based on chemical additives and the likelihood of contamination. Your selection of fish should include: bluefish, wild salmon, cod, haddock, trout, flounder, sole, hake, and red snapper. Shellfish such as lobster, shrimp, and clams should be avoided in addition to tuna and swordfish.

Your other main meals of the week should be vegetarian. However, whole-wheat products should be eaten only once or twice a week; and grains should be limited to wild rice, brown rice, spelt, and Kamut. Good substitutes for grains are sweet or white potatoes, acorn and butternut squash, or Jerusalem artichokes.

Dairy products should be substantially reduced. *All* milks (whole, skim, cow's, or goat's) should be replaced by soy or rice milk. Cottage cheese, ricotta cheese, or farmer cheese should now be eaten once or twice a week; and eggs (use the egg whites only) should be reduced to two per week.

At this point, fruits and vegetables begin to play a more prominent role in your diet. Fruit should be eaten two or three times a day between meals; or you may make an entire meal of fruits, eating, for instance, a whole cantaloupe or a large bowl of blueberries. Apples and apple juice, however, should be eliminated, as should oranges, pears, mangoes, and bananas. Alkaline fruits including watermelon, papaya, grapefruit (an acidic fruit that has alkaline properties after digestion), honeydew, and cantaloupe are preferable choices for Type A's. Tomatoes, avocados, spinach, and cabbage should be greatly reduced from salads.

You should remain at this level for about three months.

Level 4

All meats should now be completely eliminated. However, if you have difficulty making this adjustment at this level, or if you're under physical stress and still require animal protein, eat fish two or three times a week, and occasionally turkey or lamb. All lunches and dinners, barring these exceptions, should be vegetarian meals. All cheese and dairy products should also be eliminated from your diet, and eggs should be reduced to one a week.

All whole-wheat grains and wheat-derived products should now be eliminated. Only soy or sprouted-wheat products or Ezekiel bread should be eaten.

Pumpkin and sunflower seeds, almonds, walnuts, and Brazil nuts—which are all good sources of protein—should become an integral part of your diet. Eat a handful of nuts or seeds several times a day. Sprouts from alfalfa, mung beans, and adzuki beans should be incorporated into your meals because they are rich in minerals and also have high vegetable-protein content. Lima, soy, and kidney beans should be eaten for their protein. Eat a square of tofu four to five times a day.

Eat brown rice no more than twice a week, for it can be too acidic for Type A's. Also include a tablespoonful or two of olive oil on your salads or steamed vegetables every day. It has a good nutrient value and aids digestion and elimination.

This level should be worked into over a period of about four or five months, depending on how you're feeling.

Level 5

All meals should now be vegetarian, and grains and breads should be soy derived or sprouted-wheat products. You may eat one egg per week, and brown rice may be eaten once or twice a week. Dairy products should be eliminated from your diet.

Seeds, sprouts, and tofu should be eaten every day as your main sources of protein. Fruits and vegetables are now your major source of all other nutrients. This is the ideal menu for Type A's and the goal of your regimen. It should be worked into slowly, with great deliberation, and at your own pace.

Type B

Midway in characteristics between Types A and O, Type B's have a tendency to react like A's with a catarrhal nature (disposed to an inflammation of mucous membranes in the throat and nose and the production of excessive mucus) or like O's in the unbalanced state of health. An inventory of your symptoms will reveal which way the regimen will be directed.

Level 1

Regardless of your current physical tendencies, begin the program by eliminating processed and refined foods. Candy, soda, chocolate syrup, canned food, and convenience dinners should be reduced as much as possible. Replace sugar with honey, and substitute whole grains for instant and processed cereals. Introduce millet, soy/wheat, multigrains, quinoa, spelt, whole oats, or buckwheat into your diet. Substitute whole-wheat products for refined-flour products.

Reduce beef and pork as much as possible, substituting lamb, veal, turkey, or fish. Eat only soft cheeses such as buffalo mozzarella, ricotta, or raw goat's milk cheese. Replace hard alcohol with red or white wine; mix white wine half-and-half with carbonated water.

Eliminate all fried and sautéed foods. Meats and fish should be boiled or baked, organic eggs can be boiled or poached, and vegetables can be steamed.

Type B's need to exercise 30 minutes a day. The best time is in the morning. Your goal is a moderate program of activities such as jogging, swimming, hiking, bicycling, calisthenics, or hatha yoga. If your exercise program has been strenuous, reduce it now.

Stay at this level for about a month.

Level 2

Animal protein (such as veal, lamb, chicken, turkey, or fish) should be eaten once every day. Eliminate whole-wheat products and substitute them with soy products. Eat soy bread, soy-wheat cereal, Kamut, and Ezekiel bread four times a week. Add tofu squares to your meals four times a week.

Lunch should be vegetarian three times a week. Apple-cider vinegar can be used with a polyunsaturated oil (safflower or sun-flower) on salads twice a week; the other days squeeze a quarter of a lemon into the dressing. It's best to use olive oil for salads and grape-seed oil for cooking. Sea salt and kelp powder may be used in moderation as condiments.

Eat fruits three times a day between meals. Alternate steamed and raw vegetables to allow the body to adapt to the laxative effect of raw vegetables.

Start reducing your dairy products. Goat and sheep cheeses and other soft cheeses such as ricotta, cottage, or farmer cheese can be eaten four times per week. Yogurt can be eaten two or three times a week. Cut eggs back to four per week; and if you use milk, drink raw cow's or goat's milk, but limit it to two to four glasses a week. Start introducing rice and almond milk as a substitute.

Remain on this level for about two months.

Level 3

Follow one of these two diets, depending upon whether the nature of your body is catarrhal (retaining a lot of mucus) or fatigued.

Catarrhal Nature: Greatly reduce chicken from your diet. Eat veal, turkey, lamb, or buffalo once a week and fish twice a week. Recommended fish include cod, flounder, red snapper, bluefish, halibut, salmon, sea trout, and sea bass. Avoid shellfish. Your other dinners should be vegetarian—for example, a salad, steamed veg-etables, and a sweet potato or a grain such as brown rice.

188

Eliminate whole-wheat products; instead, use soy products. Greatly reduce dairy products, replacing raw cow's or goat's milk with soy milk. You may have soft cheeses once or twice a week and two eggs per week. Eat tofu four times a day.

Continue to eat fruit three times a day between meals. Apples and apple juice should be temporarily eliminated because of their high acidity level; and oranges, orange juice, bananas, and mangoes should also be avoided. Alkaline-forming fruits such as grapefruit, cantaloupe, and watermelon are better for you during this period. Lunches should be completely vegetarian.

Follow this diet for three to four months.

Fatigued Nature: Eat veal and lamb three times a week, turkey twice a week, and fish the remaining nights. Soft cheeses can be eaten two or three times a week and yogurt once a week. You may have four eggs per week. In addition, drink a glass of rice or almond milk three to four times a week.

You need to increase your protein intake: eat a square of tofu one to four times a week, and have rice protein drinks before breakfast and dinner. (Stir a tablespoon and a half of protein powder into a glass of water to make the drink.)

Whole-wheat products may be eliminated; substitute with soy products, Kamut, spelt, and Ezekiel bread. Brown rice may be eaten two to three times a week; and other grains such as buckwheat, millet, or barley may also be eaten in place of brown rice. All lunches should now be vegetarian.

Introduce olive oil into your diet to encourage proper digestion and healthy elimination. Take one tablespoon every other day, in salads, with veggies, or as is.

Reduce physical activity if your body is greatly fatigued; if not, you can exercise for an hour four times a week.

Follow this regimen for three to four months, or until you've regained your strength.

Level 4

Catarrhal Nature: Continue to eat veal and lamb once a week, and turkey and fish twice a week. Other main meals should be vegetarian.

Whole-wheat products, such as spelt bread or soy-wheat cereal, may be eaten once a week. Eat grains such as millet, barley, or buckwheat once a week. You may continue to eat brown rice once a week.

Soft cheeses may be eaten twice a week and yogurt once a week. You may have three eggs per week. Reintroduce two or three glasses of raw cow's or goat's milk per week into your diet. Soy or rice milk may be drunk as often as desired. Type B's tolerate dairy products well, but most individuals must reduce them and then reintroduce them slowly. Oranges may also be eaten once a week. Lunches should be vegetarian.

Work on this level for two to three months.

Fatigued Nature: As the fatigue abates and your body regains its strength, you may have veal once a week and lamb once every two weeks. Turkey may be eaten once or twice a week, and fish should be eaten twice a week. All other dinners should be vegetarian. (If you've noticed, I've removed chicken from the menu. Type B's should eat chicken once or twice a month.)

Soft cheeses should be consumed twice a week and yogurt once a week. Dilute whole milk with water, and eventually replace it with rice, goat's, or skim milk diluted in water, and finally, soy milk. Four eggs may be eaten per week; continue to eat tofu (about four to five times a week). Rice protein drinks should still be drunk as instructed in level 3.

Stay on this diet for two months.

Level 5

At the ideal level, Type B's can eat turkey and fish twice a week and vegetarian dinners three times a week. Every other week, substitute calf's liver, buffalo, lamb, or veal for fish or turkey. If your occupation isn't demanding, you can have meat or fish three nights a week and vegetarian four nights.

The best order of animal protein for Type B's is fish, turkey, lamb, buffalo, and beef. Choose from this selection for 12 to 14 meals a week.

Soft cheeses may be eaten twice a week and yogurt once a week. You may also eat four eggs a week.

Alternate whole-wheat and rice products: have rice products four times a week and whole-wheat products three times. You may have brown rice once or twice a week, as well as other grains such as millet or barley. Spelt is the best kind of bread for Type B's.

Apples and oranges can be eaten twice a week, but avoid bananas entirely. Sea salt and kelp powder may be eaten as desired.

Type AB

Level 1

At this initial level, eliminate processed and refined foods and those with chemical preservatives, artificial flavorings, and additives. Reduce or eliminate coffee, tea, candies, soda, syrups, and canned and instant foods. Replace bleached or enriched white-flour products with whole-wheat products. Reduce beef and pork products, gradually replacing with veal, lamb, and chicken (in moderation, you can add turkey and fish, too).

Eat only those dairy products made from raw cow's or raw goat's milk. Avoid commercially processed milk. Eggs should be from free-range hens, and use cold-pressed oil instead of commercially refined oils.

Eliminate fried or sautéed foods. Meat and fish should be grilled or baked, vegetables steamed, and eggs soft-boiled or poached. Substitute red wine for white wine. Eliminate hard alcohol and smoking as soon as possible.

Evaluate your exercise program. Your goal, like Type A's, is a calming regimen. My recommended program includes hatha yoga, tai chi, light jogging, hiking, swimming, or an aerobic workout.

Follow this level for a month or two.

Level 2

Your main meals should consist mostly of turkey, ostrich, buffalo, and fish instead of the more acidic meats like veal and lamb.

Eliminate whole-wheat products. Introduce soy products and have soy bread four times a week. Oatmeal, soy flakes, and soy granules are preferable to millet, farina, ground rice, or corn. Limit wheat germ and bran to once or twice a week.

Reduce eggs to four a week. Dilute whole milk, or substitute rice or soy milk. Soft cheeses may be eaten two or three times a week, and yogurt twice a week.

Steam your vegetables if you aren't accustomed to the laxative effect of raw vegetables. Introduce vegetarian meals at lunch (if this isn't your main meal) at least two to three times a week.

Sea salt and kelp powder may be alternated as condiments. Eliminate apple-cider vinegar; instead, use lemon juice with oil and herbs to dress vegetables or salads.

Stay at this level for up to three months.

Level 3

Completely eliminate veal from your diet. Eat turkey twice a week, fish the other nights, and lamb occasionally. Recommended fish include cod, salmon, halibut, flounder, grouper, sole, red snapper, sea or brook trout, and sea bass. Avoid shellfish, tuna, and swordfish. If possible, introduce a vegetarian night once or twice a week and start cutting back slowly on your consumption of meat and fish.

Entirely eliminate dairy products; substitute with soy products. Reduce grains such as millet, buckwheat, or barley to once every two weeks. Brown rice may be eaten once or twice a week.

Fruits and vegetables should now begin to play a prominent part in your diet. Eat fruit three or four times a day between meals. Eliminate apples and apple juice, oranges and orange juice, bananas, and mangoes. Increase vegetarian lunches to five or six per week. Vegetables may be eaten both steamed and raw. An important addition to salads at this point are sprouted seeds, including alfalfa, mung beans, lentils, and soybeans.

Take up to three months to work at this level.

Level 4

Reduce fish consumption to three times a week, and eat lamb or turkey once a week. All other dinners—and lunches—should now be vegetarian. Eliminate cheese and yogurt from your diet; replace butter with soy, safflower, or lecithin margarine. All breads should be made from soy flour.

Brown rice may be eaten once a week. Oatmeal and occasionally cornmeal, along with millet, spelt, and Ezekiel bread, may be eaten for breakfast.

Eat almonds, pumpkin seeds, and sunflower seeds every day for protein. Sprouts, which have a high mineral and protein content, should be an integral part of your daily diet. Mix them into salads or combine them with steamed vegetables. Eat lima, kidney, or soybeans for protein. One or two eggs may be eaten per week. Fruits and vegetables now make up an increasing part of your diet (in Europe, it isn't uncommon to have a plain salad for breakfast).

Work on this level for about three months.

Level 5

The ideal AB diet is vegetarian except for three or four meals a week that include a variety of fish, turkey, or lamb. All breads and grains should be rice derived, and dairy products should be avoided, although a soft cheese like mozzarella or sheep or goat cheese may be eaten once a month. Three to four eggs may be eaten per week. Eat seeds and almonds each day; and eat sprouts, an important source of protein, several times daily. You may have brown rice once a week; cereals such as oats, spelt, and Kamut every day; cornmeal twice a week; and bran once a week.

If you have a physically demanding occupation, you may want to add more fish or (occasionally) chicken to your diet to meet your energy requirements. Work into this ideal level at your own pace.

Frequently Asked Questions

This program represents a considerable departure from previous thinking and living for most people. Invariably, questions arise. Here are some of the most commonly asked questions by patients on the D'Adamo program. Hopefully, they will address some of your concerns.

1. How long will it take me to get well?
Nature works slowly but surely. If you faithfully follow your doctor's recommended menu and treatment, you will attain good health. It took years to become ill; it may take years to get better.

2. What quantity of food should I eat at each meal?
The typical stomach is the size of a fist—in most cases, people overeat. Quality, not quantity, is what's truly important. Most people should reduce their food intake and leave the table a little hungry.

3. Why do I always feel hungry?
The foods you are now eating are lighter than the cakes, pastries, meat, and gravies that you ate in the past. You should never leave the table with a bloated feeling. Overeating dulls the mind and senses, as the blood must first flow to the stomach to aid digestion for as long as it takes.

4. Why won't the menu work just by itself?

The menu has been specifically selected for your body's needs, but your body also needs cleansing and revitalizing treatments as well as herbs and vitamins to fully benefit from the menu.

5. Why do I feel tired after following my new regimen?

The body must slow down to repair itself and regenerate. Fatigue indicates that normal physical energy rather than nervous energy is being used; that is, the body is returning to a state of balance through the healing regimen that you've undertaken.

6. Can I eat at restaurants?

Grilled or baked fish, vegetables, and salads are readily available at most restaurants—so, yes, you can enjoy restaurant meals.

7. What happens when I'm invited to a house party?

Eat at home before going to a party. You'll find one or two suitable foods at any party. A word of caution: don't tell everyone about your special menu—just enjoy the company.

8. Why does my face look drawn?

This is partially due to the balancing process taking place in your body. In a short time, your face will assume an entirely healthy look.

9. Am I losing too much weight?

Most patients lose weight in the process of detoxification. Your body will determine your ideal weight. Friends may say that you've lost too much weight, but this is a normal part of the balancing process. Your weight will readjust itself to the correct level.

10. Why do I have to get up so often in the middle of the night to urinate?

Since you're drinking eight to ten glasses of water a day, as well as juices and herbal teas to revitalize your kidneys and bladder, you may have to relieve yourself during the night. Soon a healthier functioning system will result in fewer nightly bathroom visits.

11. Why do I have complaints I never had before like headaches and stomachaches?

While the body is moving into balance, periods of discomfort may occur. These periods are necessary as the energy of one organ is balanced by the energy of its counterpart. They will last a few days or a few weeks at most. Removing the symptom doesn't result in good health; removing the cause is the answer.

12. Why did I start feeling terrible as soon as I began the new regimen?

Your attitude is the most important factor. If you approach it with great distaste, you can manifest headaches and pain in your body. Don't follow the diet as if you've undertaken a task that you don't want to face. You must understand that your doctor can't cure you; you cure yourself by following his or her suggestions and letting Nature do the healing.

13. Why do my friends think I'm nuts to change my way of life?

For the most part, they're afraid to admit that their lifestyle is harmful to them, and you're doing something to positively improve yours. The best approach is not to discuss your menu and treatments with your friends. If you do, you may find that everyone is an "authority" on dieting whether or not they've been educated in the field. You should concern yourself with only one fact: you have to live in the best way suited to you. Live your own life; don't let your friends tell you how to live.

14. I read that all people should be vegetarians. Is this accurate?

Definitely not. There are many foods that aren't suitable for everyone. One man's food may be someone else's poison.

15. Are all herbal supplements beneficial?

No. Some herbs are toxic, such as quinine, digitalis (known as foxglove), and phenobarbital. The D'Adamo Institute strongly recommends nontoxic herbs and from these, only those which will energize health in your individual system. Do not take any herbs without consulting your doctor.

16. If I shouldn't have sugar, can I substitute honey?
Honey is sugar, just as white sugar is sugar.

17. Will I ever be able to drink soft drinks or carbonated drinks?
No. This is because the synthetic derivatives, sugar and carbonation, interfere with digestion and body chemistry, eventually leading to a total breakdown of the body.

18. Is there a guideline to acidic, alkaline, and neutral foods?
There might be a guideline if all people were alike. An apple is acidic for Type A's, but neutral or alkaline for Type O's. To determine what is which for whom depends upon the individual case, and for that reason, there might even be exceptions to the rule.

19. How many animal proteins can I eat at one meal? Could I have meat and fish together?
Eat one animal-protein food per meal. Also, don't combine a protein with a starch.

20. Why don't you recommend eating seafood like clams, shrimp, lobster, and mussels?
These are the scavengers of the ocean. They eat the filth off the ocean floor and are also more likely to contain higher levels of toxic mercury. Shrimp, clams, and lobster are notorious for having high levels of trans fats, which can raise your level of "bad" LDL cholesterol and increase your chance of developing coronary heart disease.

21. Can I eat fried foods?
No, because cooked oil is carcinogenic (cancer forming). Use a wok and one tablespoon of cold-pressed olive oil combined with six or seven tablespoons water, or mix water and miso for those foods you used to fry in oil. This will create a steaming effect, rather than a frying effect.

22. Why is sugar so bad for me?

During metabolism, your body uses the various vitamins, minerals, enzymes, and so on, which are stored in natural foods, to maintain and build new cells. Sugar, even so-called natural sugar, stores none of these elements. It contains only calories, which satisfy the appetite but have no nutritional value. It depletes the body reserves of many nutrients, particularly the B vitamins, and has an extreme effect on the pancreas. Sugar is truly a drug, a socially accepted one, which will ultimately upset your emotional and physical health.

23. Will my intake of vitamins ever be reduced?

As your body gains strength, your vitamin intake will be reduced. Type A's will derive the necessary vitamin supply directly from food. Types O, B, and AB will always need some vitamin supplements; in addition, Type O's will need a high-protein diet.

24. Why don't I have a strict daily menu?

Every patient should accept the responsibility for regaining health, and the first step in that direction is understanding. When you have to think through a food list and develop a menu, you're beginning to comprehend the rationale for your new regimen. Making your own decisions to regain your health is a far better procedure than having someone else tell you exactly what to do.

25. Why don't I have to count calories?

I am concerned with the chemical balance of the foods on your menu, rather than their caloric content. Weight loss, however, is quite possible with your new menu.

26. Why are you complicating my life with this new menu?

When you know which foods are good for your body, you've eliminated a source of disorder and confusion from your daily life. The foods on your menu have been selected for you on the basis of your body's requirements. All you have to do is combine them properly. You can make each meal an exciting taste discovery—invent and experiment with your menu until you do.

27. Why are you doing this to me?

I didn't create your disease—you did. What I'm doing is sharing knowledge and telling you the truth about what your body needs and wants. You must take responsibility for your health. Be patient and give it time. Realize that it took years to get sick, and it will take time to get well. If you feel that you cannot do this, *do not* attempt this menu.

CHAPTER TEN

Prevention Exercise Program

You simply cannot attain your potential for health without exercise. The human body requires movement and the proper type of exertion. Just as you create a menu according to your blood type and subtype, your exercise program has to be designed just for you. Remember that strenuous exercise is great for O's, good for B's, and detrimental to A's.

The proper type of exercise is wonderful for:

- Relieving tension
- Burning off excess calories
- Balancing blood-sugar levels
- Curbing appetite
- Increasing energy levels
- Clearing the mind
- Lowering cholesterol and triglycerides in the blood

Plan a specific exercise program and stick to it. Be selfish with your time. This is your opportunity to do something just for yourself. You're giving yourself a gift that will benefit your body, mind, and spirit. Don't let anything or anyone take it away from you.

Tip: Always warm up and cool down. Do a slow warm-up of five to ten minutes to increase circulation and bring warmth to cold, stiff tissues. Spend a few minutes shaking out your arms and legs before you begin more strenuous movements. Ankle, knee, and hip circles will lubricate the joints to prepare them for harder work. Start slowly and gradually increase effort to the desired level of exertion. End every workout with a five- to ten-minute cooldown followed by some gentle stretching. The importance of this cannot be overemphasized. Studies have shown that people who warm up and cool down adequately have fewer athletic injuries.

Type O

A demanding physical program is as vital to Type O's as their diet. O's tend to be muscular, and their blood flow is naturally sluggish. Without a vigorous exercise program to activate their blood and energy, they can become lazy and lethargic. The more that O's exercise, the more the body is stimulated, leading to an intense feeling of well-being. Jogging, gymnastics, calisthenics, hiking, swimming, and bicycling are preferred activities and should be done vigorously and on a regular basis (up to an hour a day).

In a test, athletes who were Type O were rarely fatigued after several hours of active exercise. Their bodies were charged with energy, and they were able to partake in further activities.

Whenever you start an exercise program, I suggest you start slowly and work your way up. If you are ill or exhausted, you may only be able to accomplish a few minutes a day at first. Don't be discouraged. With time and consistent effort, your ability to exercise will improve, leading you to ever-higher levels of health and fitness.

Type A

As I previously explained, Type A's function chiefly on nervous energy, so it's crucial for those who are this blood type to choose physical exercises that have a calming effect.

Jogging, calisthenics, gymnastics, or contact sports stimulate Type A bodies and will further excite them. These activities should be done with restraint. Athletes who are Type A are usually more exhausted following similar exercises because they tend to use more mental or nervous energy in their performance and consequently experience a greater general drain. After strenuous exercises, Type A's have little desire to engage in further activities or socialize.

Type A's often feel they should work off excessive nervous energy through strenuous exercise. When they do so, the immediate reaction is a feeling of relaxation, but this is due to fatigue that overwhelms the nervous system. The goal is not to achieve relief through exhaustion, but rather to calm the mind through specific exercises designed for this purpose. The best exercises for Type A's are hatha yoga, tai chi, or qi gong. Light swimming, jogging, hiking, golfing, and doubles tennis are also beneficial if done in a relaxed manner.

Type B

Exercise, which is not as vital to B's regimen as it is to A's and O's, should be done in moderation for this blood group. Whereas A's are hyperstimulated and need to be calmed and O's are often sluggish and need to be stimulated, B's bodies are moderately charged. They can jog, hike, and swim, as well as practice gymnastics, calisthenics, hatha yoga, tai chi, or qi gong for an hour several times a week. Whatever the exercise or sport, B's will find that they can simply enjoy themselves rather than work to either calm or stimulate their body.

Type AB

AB's are generally tense individuals who function primarily on nervous kinetic energy. Therefore, AB's should engage in activities that will calm and relax them while avoiding overstimulation.

Hatha yoga, tai chi, and qi gong are ideal for this. Type AB's should also participate in more strenuous exercises for five to ten minutes daily, but they must pace themselves and expend their energy economically.

Stretching

It's important to understand the basics of what you're doing before launching into any exercise program.

Anyone who has done weight training will be familiar with the concept of isolating individual muscle groups. A good weight exercise focuses on one muscle group, eliminating as many "supporting" muscle groups as possible. This guarantees that the muscle being trained will bear the brunt of the strain and can be stressed adequately using relatively lighter weights, since no supporting or contributing muscles are helping out.

The same principle applies to stretching. A good stretch isolates the muscle that is being worked and eliminates having to overcome the resistance offered by multiple muscle groups. For example, one-legged hamstring stretches are better than the two-legged kind.

Here's why: During the standard two-legged stretch (bending forward, either standing or sitting, to touch your toes) you are working against both spinal erectors (lower back), both sets of gluteus muscles (buttocks), both hamstrings, and if you grasp your toes, both calf muscles as well. This isn't particularly effective, as only the tightest muscle group will be stretched. Isolating the muscles you're trying to stretch gives you control. Since you're working against the resistance offered by only one muscle group, you can vary the intensity of the stretch from a mild pull to the point at which pain prevents you from continuing. Isolation allows focused, controlled stretching.

Stretching has beneficial effects on the muscles and joints for all blood types but is probably the most neglected part of a proper fitness program. It can significantly improve flexibility and the overall comfort of living in your body. If you're unfamiliar with stretching, it's best to learn from a qualified fitness instructor or pick up one of the many illustrated books on the subject. The following are some of the most important stretches:

The "Spinal Twist"

While seated on the floor, extend your left leg in front of you. Bend your right leg, placing your right foot on the inside of the left knee. Extend your right arm behind you to support your body. Place your left arm on the outside of the right leg. Slightly twist your torso to the right, using your left arm until you feel the stretch in your side. Hold for 10 to 30 seconds. Repeat on the other side.

Calf Stretch

Stand facing a wall, and place your left foot so that your toes are against the wall. Take a step back with your right foot. Lean forward and bend your elbows so your forearms are resting against the wall. Keeping your right foot flat on the floor, bend your left leg and shift your body forward until you feel the stretch in your calf muscle. Hold an easy stretch for 10 to 30 seconds. Do not bounce. Stretch the other leg.

Forearm Stretch

Extend your right arm out straight with the palm up. Using your left hand, pull your fingertips back toward your body until you feel the stretch in your forearm. Hold the stretch for 10 to 30 seconds. Repeat using the other arm.

Triceps Stretch

Bend your right arm so that your elbow is over and behind your head, while placing your fingers in the middle of your back. Put your left arm behind your head and pull your right elbow backward until you feel the stretch in the back of your arm. Hold it for 10 to 30 seconds. Stretch the other side.

Inner-Thigh Stretch

While seated on the floor, pull both feet inward toward the body. Grab your feet with your hands and gently lean forward while using your elbows to press downward slightly on the knees. You should feel this stretch in your inner thighs. Hold for 10 to 30 seconds.

"Cat" (Back) Stretch

This is a great way to stretch your spine. Start on your hands and knees, just like a cat. Slowly arch your back up toward the ceiling and hold in place for 10 to 30 seconds.

Hatha Yoga

Yoga is a superb form of exercise for A's, good for B's, and sufficient for O's if their subtype is A. It's one of the oldest forms of exercise known to man and is deeply rooted in the mind-body philosophy. There are many types of yoga, and while they usually share common elements, their focus is often quite different. Today, millions pack fitness studios seeking the mind-body benefits of yoga, including increased flexibility, strength, balance, and muscle tone. Unfortunately, many yoga programs in America have become too strenuous for Type A's. This is why I emphasize hatha yoga for A's, as it's a more traditional form that develops the body through the focus of the mind rather than through brute repetition of aerobic movements.

Tip: Can't get to a yoga studio or having difficulty following a book? Purchase a yoga video or DVD for beginners. It's a great introduction that allows you to try it in the privacy of your own home. While it's recommended that you find a qualified teacher to help you get started and ensure that you're performing the exercises properly, following a video or book is much better than making excuses to do nothing.

Postures

There are hundreds of yoga postures with numerous benefits, including:

- Strengthening and toning muscles
- Stretching muscles
- Improving blood circulation
- Gently exercising inner organs
- Developing concentration
- Increasing balance/equilibrium
- Increasing energy
- Calming the mind

Overall, you develop a new vitality when you practice yoga postures on a regular basis. Gradually, you may develop an awareness of your physical processes called kinesthesia. You may begin to note that your ability to control your breathing provides great relaxation to your body. By aligning the energy centers of your body (known as chakras), you begin to create more harmony and order in the functioning of the organs and systems of your body.

Yoga Suitability for Your Blood Type

Blood Type	Suitability	Number of Minutes
O	Poor	0
A	Excellent	20–60
B	Fair	10–20
AB	Good	20–60

Tai Chi

Tai chi is a Chinese martial art that is excellent for A's, good for B's, and recommended for O's who have an A subtype. Primarily practiced for its health benefits, it increases joint strength and flexibility in all areas while providing a means for dealing with tension and stress. Tai chi emphasizes complete relaxation and is essentially a form of meditation; it has even been called "meditation in motion." Although it is soft, slow, and flowing, the movements bring energy and strength to the body. Tai chi, as a form of meditation, can also help you understand yourself on a deeper level and enable you to deal with others more effectively.

Tip: Tai chi isn't as popular as yoga, but you'll be surprised how many communities offer classes, especially in medium to large urban areas. If you can't find a tai chi class, try a beginner video or check out your options online. The movements are very precise and complex, so it would be helpful to be guided by a qualified instructor.

Tai Chi Suitability for Your Blood Type

Blood Type	Suitability	Number of Minutes
O	Poor	0
A	Great	30
B	Excellent	35
AB	Great	30

Qi Gong

Similar to tai chi, qi gong springs from an ancient Chinese tradition. Practitioners believe that improving the function of *qi* (what might be called vital energy, or life force, in the West) maintains health and heals disease. In traditional Chinese medicine, good health is a result of a free-flowing, well-balanced energy system. It's believed that regular practice of qi gong cleanses the body of toxins, restores energy, reduces stress and anxiety, and helps individuals maintain a healthy and active lifestyle. It is excellent for A's, good for B's, and recommended for O's if they have the A subtype.

Tip: You might have difficulty finding a qi gong instructor. A traditional Chinese-medicine center or acupuncturist would be your best bet for locating a teacher. Videos are available if an instructor can't be found.

Qi Gong Suitability for Your Blood Type

Blood Type	Suitability	Number of Minutes
O	Poor	0
A	Great	30
B	Excellent	35
AB	Great	30

Walking

Walking is the exercise of choice for many B's, but it can be enjoyed by all blood types. When you first begin your walking program, start slowly if you're unwell or out of shape. You may at first only feel comfortable taking a five-minute stroll. That's a start. Try to go just a little bit farther on each walk.

Walking is perfect for most people in good health, regardless of age, location, or season. And there are numerous benefits: it allows you to clear your mind and relax, it forces you to breathe deeply, and it can even be done with a friend! Studies have indicated that a significant improvement in physical fitness can be achieved in just three to four weeks by walking half an hour a day, five days a week, at a pace of three miles an hour while carrying a six-and-a-half-pound load.

What to Wear

Choose comfortable walking or running shoes that are lightweight, well cushioned, and flexible across the instep. They should also have a firm heel grip and good arch support. Ideally, there should be a half-inch clearance between the end of the toes and the front of the shoes so that your toes have enough room to move freely. Wear absorbent socks, preferably a cotton or wool blend.

Safety Features

One of the most common types of accidents associated with walking is falling. A walking stick helps to prevent this mishap, gives extra support and balance, and is good exercise for the arms. When walking at night, apply reflective tape to shoes or clothes and wear light-colored clothing so that you'll be easily visible to motorists. Use common sense when walking in unknown areas, especially at night. Always carry identification and an emergency phone number, plus any medical alerts in case of an emergency.

Tips: Walk with a friend. You can encourage each other, especially on those days when you may be tempted to skip exercising because you're too tired or stressed. These are the times when you need to exercise even more! Fatigue and stress can be alleviated through appropriate exercise. If you don't have a friend who's available to walk with you on a regular basis, then walk with your dog or listen to music.

Don't overdo it. Create a moderate exercise schedule to start with and slowly build up. For example, at first it may be one day on, one day off. Don't be too hard on yourself. Most of all, enjoy yourself.

Walking Suitability for Your Blood Type

Blood Type	Suitability	Number of Minutes
O	Fair	35–60
A	Good	5–10
B	Good	30
AB	Excellent	10–20

Aerobic Exercise

Aerobic exercise promotes cardiovascular fitness by raising your heart rate to a targeted level for 20 or more continuous minutes. You can become adept at gauging your level of exertion without counting your pulse. You should notice that you're breathing more deeply but not working so hard that you couldn't carry on a conversation. These exercises strengthen your heart and allow it to pump more blood with each beat. In addition, aerobic exercise improves the capacity of the lungs, helps control weight, and increases muscle and joint flexibility, making you less susceptible to injury. Common examples include power walking, jogging/running, swimming, rowing, stair climbing, bicycling, cross-country skiing, step and dance exercise classes, and roller-skating. Sports or activities that tend to stop and go, such as tennis, calisthenics, racquetball, and basketball are *not* considered good cardiovascular exercises because they don't raise the pulse rate high enough, nor are they capable of sustaining an increased pulse rate over a period of time.

Perform this type of exercise only if your doctor has recommended it for you.

Aerobic Suitability for Your Blood Type

Blood Type	Suitability	Number of Minutes
O	Excellent	No limit
A	Poor	0
B	Good	5–30
AB	Poor	0–5

Aqua Fitness

Swimming is one of the best ways to get a total body workout. It has cardiovascular, strengthening, and flexibility components that are essential parts of being fit. The biggest advantage of swimming as a form of exercise is that water's buoyancy reduces a person's "weight" by 90 percent. Therefore, weight-bearing muscles, bones, and joints have less stress put upon them; and circulation to congested areas is improved.

Ideas for Your Water Workout

- Water walking or running offers a cardiovascular workout and strength training (from water resistance). Simply stand in waist-deep water and move forward, sideways, or backward to work different muscle groups.

- For another aerobic exercise, tread water or "run" in deep water while wearing a life jacket to keep your head out of the water. As you become stronger, you may be able to do this without a life jacket.

- Use aquatic equipment to intensify your workout. These are available at many public pools and sporting-goods stores. For example, use a kickboard to strengthen your legs or hand paddles to target your arms.

Aqua-Fitness Suitability for Your Blood Type

Blood Type	Suitability	Number of Minutes
O	Good	10–20
A	Good	0–15
B	Excellent	10–20
AB	Good	0–20

Jogging/Running

For the O blood type, running is probably the best workout, as it delivers the most benefits per minute of exercise. It's also good for B's but should be strictly avoided by A's, as it exhausts the body. Running is only appropriate if an individual's knees and other joints can handle the stress. Running on trails or dirt roads reduces the impact and often provides a more peaceful setting in which to exercise.

Getting started and staying motivated can be difficult. Like walking, jogging can be done anytime, anywhere; and it involves only one person. In addition, it has all the health benefits of walking and more: it conditions the heart, improves muscle tone and strength, relieves stress, and can help with a variety of health problems. While walking may conjure up all the pleasures of a casual stroll, jogging requires more of a commitment to training.

Once you're past the initial discomfort, you may find it to be the most rewarding and natural of all exercises. It takes discipline to run, but the benefits are measurable improvements in endurance and strength. It also delivers a wonderful sense of peace. The following are basic steps to starting a running program.

Running Guidelines

Warm up first by shaking out the limbs and doing joint circles as described earlier. Proceed with either a fast walk or a slow jog and then gradually build up to a pace that's comfortable for

213

you. Stay as relaxed as possible while running. Keep your back straight and your shoulders back. Let your arms swing naturally while keeping your shoulders very relaxed. Many runners tend to hunch up the shoulders, which makes them tense and sore. When you come to a hill, it's only natural to lean forward a bit, which is perfectly fine.

Don't worry about how far you're going. Rather than set a distance goal, set a time goal and increase your time gradually. Experts recommend an increase of only 5 to 10 percent a week to avoid burnout or injury from overexertion.

Finally, bring some cool water along to prevent your body from becoming dehydrated.

Running Suitability for Your Blood Type

Blood Type	Suitability	Number of Minutes
O	Excellent	60+
A	Poor	0
B	Good	15–30
AB	Fair	10

❧ ❧ ❧

CHAPTER ELEVEN

Prevention Recipes

The following recipes are designed to help you get started with the program. As you become more familiar with the specific foods in your diet plan, you can adapt these recipes by substituting ingredients (such as meats, fish, vegetables, herbs, and spices) from your diet sheet for those that aren't recommended for your blood type. Be creative and experiment. With a little time, energy, and determination, your meals will become an adventure in eating. Above all, remember that as you explore your healthy new menu, you're combining the pleasure of eating with the knowledge that you're greatly improving your well-being.

I want to acknowledge the contributions of these recipes from many patients, family members, and friends, including Bruce and Maria Martino, Nancy Limberger, Antonio and Antonietta Mucciarone, Robert and Jennifer Henley, Benedetta Del Sorbo, Jennifer Henley, Faith Backus Lyons, Christiana D'Adamo, and Michele D'Adamo.

Soups

Homemade soups are wonderfully nutritious. They initially take some time to prepare but provide many convenient, on-the-go meals. A simple vegetarian soup base can be turned into various dishes if you add some meat or tofu that you happen to have in the refrigerator on a given day. I recommend that you freeze soups in small individual containers so that you'll always have a meal handy if you're tired or pressed for time. Here are some delicious soup and stock recipes.

CELERY SOUP

3 cloves garlic, minced
8 celery stalks, chopped
½ onion, diced
2 tsp. curry powder
    or fresh parsley
2 Tbsp. mustard
1 Tbsp. white miso (diluted)
Sea salt (to taste)

On low heat, sauté garlic, celery, and onion in a pot in about 1cm water. Bring to a boil, stir in mustard and curry (or parsley), and then reduce heat and simmer 5 to 7 minutes or until celery is tender. In a separate dish, dilute white miso with some of the soup. Add the diluted white miso to the pot and season with salt. You can serve it as is, or add the ingredients to a blender for a creamy soup or as a sauce over vegetables.

DAIKON CONSOMMÉ

1L water
150g thickly sliced daikon
1–2 Tbsp. lemon juice
1–2 green onions, thinly sliced for a garnish

In a soup pot, bring water to a boil. Add daikon, cover, and simmer on low heat until the daikon is tender (about 7 to 10 minutes). Remove from heat and season to taste with lemon. Serve with green onions. If you prefer a smoother soup, add the mixture to a food processor or blender and puree to desired consistency.

FISH STEW

2 tsp. grape-seed oil
2 small leeks, minced
Sea salt
1–2 Tbsp. fresh basil
1 daikon, cubed
75g Jerusalem artichokes, cubed
    (add swede, turnips, or both, if desired)
2 carrots, chopped into 1cm pieces
720ml soy milk or rice milk
450g haddock or other firm white-fleshed fish,
    cut up into pieces
Fresh parsley, minced (for garnish)

Heat oil in a pot over medium heat; then add leeks, a pinch of sea salt, and basil, stirring until the leeks begin to soften (about 3 minutes). Add daikon, Jerusalem artichokes (and turnips and/ or swede), and carrots. Cook for about a minute. Add soy or rice milk, and bring to a boil. Cover and reduce heat, cooking until vegetables are just tender (about 10 minutes). Add fish and simmer uncovered until vegetables are soft in the center (about 10 minutes). Season to taste with sea salt, and simmer 5 to 7 minutes; garnish with parsley.

LENTIL SOUP

1 tsp. grape-seed oil
1 onion, diced
1 small leek, diced
1 celery stalk, diced
1 carrot, diced
100g lentils, rinsed well
1.2L water
1 piece kombu (a type of seaweed),
   soaked in warm water
1 tsp. or less saffron
Sea salt (to taste)
Juice and grated peel of one lemon
30g tofu croutons (see recipe at the end
   of this section)

Heat oil in soup pot over medium heat. Add onion and leek and cook 4 minutes. Add celery and carrot, and cook an additional 4 minutes. Top with lentils and stir briefly, just enough to coat the lentils with oil. Add water and kombu, and bring to a boil. Cover and cook over low heat until lentils are soft (about 35 minutes). Season to taste with saffron and sea salt, and simmer 20 more minutes. Remove from heat, and stir in grated lemon peel and juice. Garnish with several tofu croutons per bowl.

PUMPKIN SOUP

1 pumpkin
1.5L vegetable broth (you can use the vegetable
   stock recipe in this chapter, if you wish)
1 tsp. cinnamon
100g celery, minced
A pinch of garlic, minced
Basil (to taste)

Scoop out the seeds from the pumpkin. Fill the pumpkin with vegetable broth, cinnamon, celery, garlic, and basil. Bake in a 180°C oven until flesh inside the pumpkin is tender. Serve the soup directly from the pumpkin at the table. This makes a very attractive centerpiece for a fall meal.

CREAMY SQUASH SOUP

600g squash, sliced
1 large onion, sliced
1.5L water or vegetable stock
2 Tbsp. grape-seed oil
1 tsp. sea salt
Parsley, chopped (to garnish)

Combine all of the ingredients except parsley in a large pot, and simmer for 30 minutes. Using a food processor or blender, puree the mixture until creamy. Garnish with chopped parsley.

VEGETARIAN SOUP

Assorted vegetables, chopped (use veggies that
   are recommended for your blood type)
1 clove garlic
1 Tbsp. olive oil

In a large pot, combine vegetables, olive oil, and garlic. (Set some chopped vegetables aside to incorporate into the soup later, if desired.) Sauté on a low flame until veggies are cooked. Remove from the stove and puree the mixture. Return mixture to the pot and heat over a low flame, while adding water as needed to thin the mixture and obtain the desired souplike consistency. Add remaining chopped vegetables, and simmer until they're fully cooked.

(Depending upon your blood type, you can add meat, fish, or tofu. You can also experiment with this soup base by adding beans, rice, or pasta and various herbs and spices.)

WINTER-VEGETABLE SOUP

1 tsp. grape-seed oil
1 leek, halved, well-rinsed, and cut into 2.5cm
   pieces
1 piece of kombu
150g winter squash (or butternut or acorn
   squash), cubed
1 small sweet potato, cubed
2 carrots, chopped into small pieces and boiled
150g daikon, diced
1.2L vegetable stock (the recipe is in the
   next section)
2–3 tsp. white miso
75g white cannellini beans, cooked
175g broccoli florets
1–2 green onions, thickly sliced (to garnish)

Heat oil in a large pot over medium heat and add leek, cooking for about 2 minutes. Add kombu, squash, sweet potato, carrots, and daikon; then slowly add stock. Bring to a boil, and then reduce heat to low and cover. Cook for 35 to 40 minutes. Put a small amount of stock in a separate dish, and add white miso, stirring until dissolved. Stir white-miso mixture into soup, add beans and broccoli florets, and simmer until the broccoli turns bright green (about 4 minutes). Serve and garnish with green onions.

MARINATED TOFU/TOFU CROUTONS
(To be used in soups and salads)

450g firm or extra-firm tofu, sliced 0.5cm thick
240ml grape-seed oil
Juice of ½ lemon
Sea salt (to taste)
2 cloves garlic, crushed
⅛ tsp. chilli paste with garlic
1 tsp. oregano

Mix all of the ingredients to make a marinade, and fully immerse the tofu for two to three hours. Place marinated tofu on an oiled baking sheet, and bake at 200°C for 30 to 40 minutes. To make croutons, cut the tofu in cubes before baking.

TURKEY OR BUFFALO MEATBALLS
(To be used in soups)

450g ground turkey or buffalo
1 tsp. garlic, minced
1 tsp. dried parsley flakes
1 Tbsp. safflower or sunflower oil
2 Tbsp. almond meal (optional)
1 tsp. fresh or dried sage (optional)

Mix ingredients together in a large bowl and shape into 2cm diameter balls. Bake on a baking sheet (uncovered) at 200°C for approximately 15 minutes.

Stocks

Use stocks as the foundation for soups and stews.

ONION STOCK

2 tsp. grape-seed oil
5–6 onions, thinly sliced
1 leek, diced
Sea salt (to taste)
2.5L water
3 celery stalks, sliced
2 bay leaves
Parsley sprigs

Heat oil in a large pot over medium heat. Add onions, diced leek, and a pinch of sea salt and cook, stirring occasionally until onions are translucent and fragrant (about 5 minutes). Add a small amount of water and simmer over low heat for 15 minutes. Add remaining water and other ingredients, and bring soup to a boil. Reduce heat to low, and simmer uncovered (about 1 hour). Strain the stock, pressing out the liquid. Discard the solids.

TURKEY STOCK

1 turkey carcass (organic)
1 bay leaf
½ tsp. dried marjoram leaves
½ tsp. dried thyme leaves
½ tsp. dried basil leaves
1 medium-sized onion, chopped
50g celery, chopped
75g carrots, sliced
Sea salt (to taste)

Remove any meat from carcass, and set aside for later use. Break up carcass, cracking large bones. Place bones in a large pot. Add remaining ingredients and enough cold water to cover. Bring stock to a boil. Reduce heat, cover, and simmer for 3 hours. Let stock cool slightly; then strain. Store stock in refrigerator, and skim off fat before using.

VEGETABLE STOCK

1 onion, sliced
1 Tbsp. grape-seed or walnut oil
Spring onions (several)
1 leek, sliced
2–3 garlic cloves, unpeeled
Sea salt (to taste)
2.5L water
2 carrots, sliced
2 bay leaves
Parsley, basil, rosemary, oregano, or thyme;
    tie herbs together with a string

Sauté sliced onion in a pot, in a little oil. Add the rest of the ingredients, and bring to a boil. Reduce heat and simmer, uncovered, for about an hour. Put stock through strainer, pressing as much liquid as you can from the vegetables before discarding them.

Salads

Salads are quick to put together and usually travel well. Here are a few combinations and salad-dressing suggestions.

BABY-ARTICHOKE SALAD

12 fresh baby artichokes
Juice of ½ lemon
¼ tsp. sea salt
4 cloves garlic, pressed
1 tsp. dried oregano
1 Tbsp. mustard (optional)
80ml olive oil
1 Tbsp. fresh Italian parsley, finely chopped

Bring a large pot of salted water to a boil. With a sharp knife, cut off the artichoke stems and remove the top inch or so from each artichoke. Boil the artichokes for 20 minutes or until it's easy to pull the leaves off with your fingers. Drain well. While the artichokes are cooking, make the dressing by combining all of the remaining ingredients. As soon as the artichokes are drained, toss them gently with the dressing. Marinate from 2 hours to overnight. Serve the artichokes in the dressing.

BROCCOLI SALAD

525g broccoli buds, steamed
25g green onions, diced
1 Tbsp. fresh basil
Vegetable salt (to taste)
Lemon and olive-oil dressing

Combine all of the ingredients and toss with lemon and oil dressing.

INSALATA DI RISO

110g brown rice
4 Roma tomatoes
4–5 black olives, chopped
2 tsp. capers
2–3 fresh basil leaves, finely chopped
1 Tbsp. extra-virgin olive oil
Sea salt (to taste)
Lemon juice (to taste)

Add rice to salted boiling water, and cook for 30 minutes in a pressure cooker. Dip tomatoes in the water for 30 seconds and peel them. Cut them in half, remove seeds, and dice; then place them in a large bowl. Add olives, capers, basil, olive oil, and sea salt; mix well. Set aside until rice is done cooking. Fluff rice and add it to the bowl with other ingredients. Mix well, add lemon juice, and serve. If prepared in advance, serve at room temperature and add lemon juice at the last minute.

SPINACH SALAD

Baby spinach
Frozen peas or fresh mangetout
Pesto (see the Basil Pesto recipe in the
    following section)
Toasted pine nuts

Toss all ingredients together. If you have a lot left over, put it in a blender with a little broth or water and turn it into sauce for veggies.

BLENDED HERB DRESSING

1 tsp. each of fresh savory, parsley, tarragon,
  and dill, minced
1 egg yolk
110ml olive oil
15g watercress, chopped
2 Tbsp. green onions, chopped
2 Tbsp. lemon juice

Blend all the ingredients until well mixed. Chill before serving.

NATURAL HERB DRESSING

1 tsp. each of aniseed, dill weed, spearmint,
  and tarragon
1 clove garlic, pressed
300ml olive oil
160ml lemon juice

Crush the herbs into a fine paste. Add garlic, oil, and lemon juice to the mixture; and shake well. Refrigerate before serving.

TOFU-HERB DRESSING

1 square of tofu
1 to 2 cloves of garlic
2 Tbsp. fresh dill
2 Tbsp. fresh Italian parsley
Juice of ½ lemon
60–120ml water
Olive oil

Add ingredients to a blender or food processor, and slowly drizzle in oil while blending until you get the desired consistency. Blend until well mixed. Chill before serving.

Appetizers and Side Dishes

Who said you can't have a great appetizer on this meal program? Here are a few ideas to whet your appetite.

ARTICHOKE ITALIANO

3 artichokes
25g fresh parsley
5 cloves garlic
120ml olive oil
120ml chicken broth
120ml water
Sea salt (to taste)

Cut tops and bottoms from artichokes. Pull off petals and place hearts in a gallon pan with lid. Add all the other ingredients, and cook until tender at a high heat.

ROCKET PESTO

150g chopped rocket, include stems
25g walnuts, chopped
3 cloves garlic, minced
5g fresh basil
120ml olive oil
½ Tbsp. white miso

Combine all ingredients except olive oil and white miso in a food processor and chop until coarse. While machine is running, drizzle olive oil and then white miso, mixing until combined. Serve over spelt pasta or add to steamed vegetables.

ASPARAGUS SAUTÉ

450g thin stalks of asparagus, chopped into
   2.5cm to 4cm pieces
4–6 shiitake mushrooms (wash and remove
   stems); thinly sliced (0.5cm thick)
2 Tbsp. grape-seed oil

Heat oil in skillet over medium heat. Add asparagus and mushrooms, and lower heat to medium-low. Stir frequently until asparagus pieces soften (about 10 minutes).

ASPARAGUS SPEAR FRIES

1 bunch of asparagus, trimmed with woody
   ends cut off
Olive oil
Sea salt
Pepper

Preheat oven to 200°C.Place asparagus on a baking sheet and coat lightly with olive oil. Sprinkle with sea salt (lightly) and pepper. Bake for 10 minutes and remove from the oven, turning the asparagus over for equal browning. Bake for another 5 minutes or until the asparagus is crispy at the tips.

BASIL PESTO

50g fresh basil (lightly packed)
2 cloves garlic
110ml olive oil
50g walnuts or pine nuts (optional)

Blend ingredients in a blender or food processor. Toss with freshly steamed vegetables.

GARLIC HUMMUS

1 can chickpeas
2 Tbsp. roasted garlic (use "Michele's Famed
   Roasted Garlic" recipe)
1 Tbsp. olive oil
Juice of ½ lemon
¼ to ½ tsp. dried oregano

Add all ingredients to a food processor and blend until smooth.
If mixture is too thick, add a small amount of oil until the desired
consistency is reached. Heat on low and serve.

KALE AND ONION STIR-FRY

1 bunch of kale
Sunflower oil (enough to coat wok)
2 onions, sliced
2 Tbsp. lemon juice
1 Tbsp. wheat-free tamari

Clean kale and remove ribs. Put a little bit of oil in wok, heat
on high, and add kale and onions, stirring for 1 to 2 minutes. Add
lemon juice and tamari, reduce heat, and simmer until onions are
tender.

CREAMED KALE OR DANDELION GREENS

2 bunches of kale or dandelion greens
1–2 Tbsp. wheat-free tamari
60ml to 80ml tahini

Steam greens until tender. While greens are still warm, add
tamari and tahini (this can be done in a pan over low heat). Stir
well until smooth. You may need to add a bit of water to blend
tahini. Adjust tamari to taste.

MICHELE'S FAMED ROASTED GARLIC

4 garlic heads
2 tsp. grape-seed oil
Sea salt (to taste)

Heat oven to 180°C. Peel a bit of the paper skin from around each head of garlic, leaving just enough to hold the cloves together. Cut 0.5cm from the top of each bulb to expose the cloves. Place heads in a cake pan or cookie sheet. Drizzle oil on each and sprinkle with sea salt. Bake for 45 to 50 minutes or until garlic is tender. Cool slightly. To serve, gently squeeze one end of each clove to release the roasted garlic. Spread on spelt bread, rice crackers, or veggies. (It's great on meat, too!)

TOFU-OLIVE DIP

60ml grape-seed oil
3–4 cloves garlic, minced
225g firm tofu, boiled 5 minutes and drained
   (boiling makes it smooth, not grainy)
Juice from one lemon
Sea salt (a pinch to taste)
5–6 green olives, pitted and minced
50g capers, drained (optional)

Heat oil in a small skillet over medium heat. Add garlic and cook until fragrant (1 to 2 minutes). Place tofu, oil with garlic, lemon juice, and sea salt into a food processor; and puree until smooth. Transfer into a mixing bowl, and gently fold in green olives and capers. Chill and serve with crackers or vegetables.

TOFU PÂTÉ

450g soft tofu
2 tsp. umeboshi paste (optional)
1 tsp. tahini
2–3 green onions, minced
1–2 celery stalks, diced
1 carrot, boiled and grated
5g fresh parsley, minced
Juice of one lemon

Bring a pot of water to a boil, add tofu, cook for 1 to 3 minutes. Drain tofu and blend in a food processor with umeboshi paste and tahini until smooth. Fold in onions, celery, grated carrot, parsley, and lemon juice. Chill, then serve with rice crackers, celery sticks, or other vegetables that need a little extra zest.

Entrées

CHICKEN OREGANO

1 chicken, cut into quarters
2 cloves garlic, minced
1 bunch of parsley, chopped
½ Tbsp. dried, crushed oregano (this is a strong-
    flavored herb, so you may want to experiment
    with the quantity)
2–3 Tbsp. olive oil
Sea salt, a pinch (optional)
Juice of one large lemon

Preheat oven to 190°C. In a bowl, combine garlic, parsley, oregano, olive oil, sea salt, and lemon juice. Massage mixture into chicken quarters; and place chicken, skin side up, in a shallow roasting pan. Pour remainder of mixture over chicken and marinate for approximately 20 minutes. Roast in oven for 1 to 1½ hours, depending on size of chicken. Internal temperature should read 82°C.

CHILEAN SEA BASS WITH LEMONGRASS

550g Chilean sea bass, cut in chunks; skin and
bones removed

1–2 tsp. grape-seed oil

Several cloves of garlic, peeled and crushed

Fresh ginger, peeled and minced (about a
thumb-size piece)

4 to 5 medium tomatoes (or 12 to 15 cherry
tomatoes), chopped

1 stalk of lemongrass, cut into 15cm pieces

100g celery, shredded

150g carrots, shredded

240–720ml water

Sea salt (to taste)

Heat the oil in a large saucepan. Add garlic, ginger, tomatoes, and lemongrass. Cook until the tomatoes are mushy. Add the celery, carrots, and 240ml of water. Cook for 10 to 15 minutes, until mixture is bubbling. Add fish chunks. (If necessary, add more water until there's just enough to cover the fish.) Cover pan and poach until the fish is cooked (about 20 minutes). Remove any pieces of lemongrass, and add sea salt to taste. The flavors become enhanced with aging. Put in the refrigerator, and have it for breakfast or lunch the next day.

CHINESE-STYLE STEAMED FISH

550g halibut, cut into 4 pieces

3 green onions, cut into 7.5cm pieces

150g fresh mushrooms, sliced

6 leaves of cabbage, sliced into 10cm pieces

2 slices fresh gingerroot, finely chopped

2 cloves garlic, chopped

60ml wheat-free tamari

30ml water

Arrange half of the green onions at the bottom of the steamer, and add half of the mushrooms and cabbage pieces on top of the onions. Place fish on top of the cabbage, and sprinkle with gingerroot and garlic. Place remaining vegetables on top of fish. Drizzle tamari and water over everything. Place steaming basket in 2.5cm of water, and cover. Steam for 15 to 20 minutes or until fish flakes easily.

CITRUS FISH

225g whitefish or grouper
60ml fresh lime juice
1 tsp. tarragon leaves
40g chopped onion

Place fish in a baking dish; and add lime juice, tarragon, and onion. Bake at 160°C for 15 to 20 minutes.

HERB-CRUSTED FISH

450g flounder, sole, or grouper
2 egg whites
5g chopped fresh herbs: parsley,
    basil, rosemary, sage, or dill
2 garlic cloves, minced
¼ tsp. sea salt
Grape-seed oil
Juice of ½ lemon

Rinse fish fillets in cold water and pat dry with a paper towel. Beat the egg whites in a shallow bowl. Spread herbs, garlic, and sea salt on a plate. Dip fillets in egg whites and then in the herb mixture, pressing the herbs onto the fish. Coat skillet with oil, and add fillets. Cook over medium heat for 3 to 4 minutes on each side until the fish is cooked through. Squeeze lemon juice on each fillet right before serving.

Variation: Steam fish with herbs without using egg whites.

HERB-MARINATED OSTRICH STEAK

450g ostrich
60ml oil
2½ Tbsp. garlic, finely chopped
1 Tbsp. fresh rosemary, crushed
1 Tbsp. fresh thyme (leaves)
½ tsp. sea salt

In a bowl, mix together all of the ingredients (except for the ostrich meat). Add meat, turning to coat well. Cover the bowl securely, and marinate in the refrigerator for an hour, turning occasionally. Remove meat from marinade (and discard the marinade). Place on rack in grill pan so that the surface of the meat is three to four inches from heat. Grill 26 to 31 minutes for medium-rare to medium doneness, turning once. Carve into slices.

LAMB SHISH KEBABS

550g lamb cubes, 2.5cm cubes
2 Tbsp. fresh coriander, minced (optional)
1 tsp. ground cumin
1 tsp. paprika (optional)
2–3 large garlic cloves, smashed
120ml grape-seed oil
8 mushrooms
2 medium onions, quartered
1 courgette, cubed

Mix coriander, cumin, paprika, and garlic with oil, making it into a paste. Rub seasoning on lamb cubes. Thread the ingredients on skewers alternating lamb, onion, and vegetables. Grill directly over medium heat for 6 to 8 minutes. Remove from grill, and let sit for a few minutes before serving.

(You can use any other vegetables you like; for instance, leeks and fennel are great options.)

LEMON CHICKEN

900g chicken pieces
½ tsp. dried thyme
60ml lemon juice
½ tsp. dried rosemary
½ tsp. celery salt
1 small onion, chopped
4 Tbsp. grape-seed oil

Arrange chicken pieces in a single layer in a baking dish. Mix together remaining ingredients and pour over chicken. Marinate for one hour. Cover and bake at 160°C for 45 minutes to an hour. This dish may be prepared up to one day in advance and refrigerated until ready to cook.

RACK OF LAMB

½ rack (4 little chops per person); or 1 rack New
   Zealand baby lamb (serves 2 people per rack)
1 Tbsp. Dijon mustard
2 Tbsp. fresh rosemary, chopped
1 clove garlic, crushed

Preheat oven to 220°C. Remove most of the fat from the lamb, cut rack in half, and rub Dijon mustard all over the meaty part. Combine rosemary and garlic on a flat plate, and dip mustard-covered rack into mixture, covering meat as evenly as possible. Let stand at room temperature for 15 to 20 minutes, allowing meat to marinate. In a shallow baking dish, place the rack halves in a standing position opposite each other (using rack bones for support), and roast in oven (18 minutes for medium).

ROASTED CHICKEN WITH ROSEMARY

1 chicken, about 2.25kg
4 branches fresh rosemary
2 celery stalks, cut into large pieces
1 carrot, chopped
4 whole garlic cloves, peeled
1 Tbsp. olive oil
Sea salt (optional)
½ lemon

Preheat oven to 180°C. Stuff the chicken with 2 branches of rosemary, celery, carrot, and garlic; and truss the legs. Massage chicken with olive oil and sprinkle with sea salt. Tuck remaining 2 branches of rosemary under wings. (The rosemary will burn slightly during the roasting process, which will intensify flavors.) Roast in the oven approximately 1½ hours. The internal temperature should read 82°C. After removing from oven, squeeze lemon juice over chicken, and let it sit for a few minutes. Remove strings, stuffing, and rosemary prior to carving and serving.

ROASTED HERB AND TOMATO LAMB CHOPS

12 lamb chops, trimmed of excess fat
10g chopped fresh mint
10g chopped fresh dill
10g chopped fresh basil
10g grape-seed oil
4 cloves garlic, chopped
80ml vegetable stock
4 tomatoes, peeled and chopped (optional)
Sea salt (to taste)

Preheat oven to 260°C. Lightly rub some of the herbs on the lamb chops, and season with sea salt. In a large skillet over high heat, add the oil and sear the chops on one side. Roast it in the oven for a few minutes until medium rare. Remove to warm plates. In the same skillet on the stove, add the garlic, stock, and tomatoes. Bring to a quick boil, and add the rest of the herbs. Adjust seasoning as needed. Spoon some of the herbs and tomatoes over the lamb chops and serve.

ROASTED LEG OF LAMB

1 bone-in leg of lamb, about 2.25kg
Garlic cloves (several), slivered
1 bunch of parsley, chopped
Sea salt to taste (optional)

Preheat oven to 160°C. Place lamb into roasting dish. With a sharp knife, make several small slits into meat, and place a sliver of garlic and a good pinch of parsley in each of the slits. Rub a little sea salt all over the leg, and roast until meat thermometer reads an internal temperature of 75°C (for medium rare, about 1½ hours). When done cooking, remove from oven and let sit for a few minutes before carving.

ROASTED TURKEY

1 turkey, 8–9kg
2 large onions, quartered
1 bay leaf
1 dried thyme sprig
2 cloves garlic
225g of the Institute's Spread (110g sweet butter, 60ml grape-seed or olive oil, 1 vitamin E capsule, and 1 lecithin capsule; whip together and refrigerate)

Preheat oven to 180°C. Place onions, bay leaf, thyme, and garlic in the cavity of the turkey. Lightly oil roasting pan with the

Institute's Spread (or the recommended oil for your blood type). Heat pan in the oven until it's hot (about 5 minutes). Place turkey on its side in hot roasting pan. Roast 40 minutes, basting occasionally. Turn turkey breast side up.

Continue to roast, basting frequently until meat thermometer inserted in the thickest part of thigh registers 77°C. This should take another hour and 40 minutes or so. When ready, transfer turkey to a heated serving platter. Remove onions, bay leaf, thyme, and garlic from cavity before carving.

SALMON STEAK

1 salmon steak
1 tsp. grape-seed oil
2 Tbsp. fresh mint
1 small garlic clove, minced
½ tsp. dried oregano
¼ tsp. sea salt (optional)
1 small courgette, halved lengthwise, then sliced
  crosswise 0.5cm thick

Preheat oven to 220°C. Place salmon in a small baking dish; drizzle with ¼ tsp. oil. In a small bowl, stir together mint, garlic, oregano, and sea salt. Sprinkle half the mixture over both sides of the salmon. Bake until opaque throughout (about 10 minutes). As the salmon bakes, heat remaining oil in a skillet over medium heat. Add courgette, tossing occasionally until tender (6 to 8 minutes). Stir in the remaining mixture of mint, garlic and oregano. Serve with salmon.

SESAME TOFU

900g firm tofu, cubed
80ml wheat-free tamari
60ml grape-seed oil

2 cloves garlic, minced
1 Tbsp. gingerroot, grated
125g sesame seeds, ground

Combine tamari, oil, garlic, and gingerroot. Marinate the tofu in the mixture for 2 hours. Roll the tofu in the ground sesame seeds, and bake on an oiled cookie sheet for 15 minutes at 180°C.

SOLE WITH ALMONDS

Grape-seed oil (enough to grease pan)
450g sole or other lean fish fillet
35g sliced almonds or chopped walnuts
1½ Tbsp. grated lemon peel
1½ Tbsp. lemon juice
½ tsp. sea salt
½ tsp. paprika

Heat oven to 190°C. Grease the bottom of the baking sheet with oil. Cut the fish fillet into four servings, and place the pieces (skin side down) in the greased pan. In a small bowl, mix the nuts, lemon peel, lemon juice, sea salt, and paprika. Spoon the mixture over the fish. Bake uncovered for 15 to 20 minutes or until the fish flakes easily with a fork.

TOFU STEAK

450g extra-firm tofu, pressed
4 Tbsp. wheat-free, low-sodium tamari
1 tsp. grated ginger
1 large clove of garlic, crushed
1 Tbsp. spelt flour
Grape-seed oil for sautéing
2 Tbsp. toasted sesame seeds
2 Spring onions, sliced (for garnish)

Press tofu for 15 minutes (wrap in a dry cloth, place a cutting board on it, and apply weight, such as a teakettle or other pot filled with water). Mix together tamari, ginger, and garlic; and set aside. Remove tofu from cloth, and cut in half lengthwise to produce two flat rectangles. Dip each one in spelt flour, gently shaking off excess. Heat the oil in a pan. Sauté tofu slices over medium heat for several minutes, lightly browning both sides. Reduce heat and poke holes in the slices with a fork. Generously brush tofu with tamari mixture, allowing the liquid to penetrate. Brown bottom of the slices, then turn over and brush remainder of the tamari mixture on tofu and cook a few minutes more. Serve tofu steak brown side up, and sprinkle with sesame seeds and sliced spring onions.

TOFU STIR-FRY WITH VEGETABLES

450g extra-firm tofu, cubed
2 Tbsp. wheat-free, low-sodium tamari
2 cloves garlic, crushed
1 tsp. grated ginger
120ml low-sodium vegetable broth
2 Tbsp. grape-seed oil
250g mixed vegetables of your choice
30g toasted almonds, sliced

In a wok, combine tamari, garlic, ginger, and vegetable broth; and bring to a boil. Add tofu cubes, cover, and simmer for 7 minutes. Remove tofu and remaining liquid from wok. Heat oil in wok and stir-fry vegetable mixture over medium heat for 5 minutes. Add tofu and liquid, and mix thoroughly until heated through. Sprinkle with toasted almonds. (Trade the tofu for buffalo, turkey, or beef; it's just as delicious.)

TURKEY-TOFU BURGER

⅔ block soft or firm plain tofu
1 stalk celery, finely chopped
Salt and garlic (to taste)
1 tsp. turmeric
2 Tbsp. safflower or sunflower oil
900g ground turkey

In a large bowl, mash the tofu into small pieces. Add chopped celery, salt, garlic, turmeric, and oil; mix well. Stir in the ground turkey until well blended. Form into two or three small balls (enough to fill the palm of your hand), and place on a baking sheet. Press in flat rounds about 2cm thick. Grill on each side until golden brown. This recipe makes about 12 burgers and can be prepared ahead and frozen. They also pack well when traveling and can be cut out into bite-size pieces and reheated nicely.

Variations: Chopped onions, coriander, or fresh garlic may be added or substituted in the mixture. Other spices such as thyme, sage, and rosemary can be substituted as seasonings.

TURKEY WRAPS

Soy wraps
Garlic hummus (can purchase organic or use the
   recipe in the previous section)
Turkey slices (organic)
½ cucumber, thinly sliced
50g alfalfa sprouts

Lay soy wraps out flat, and lightly spread garlic hummus. Add alfalfa sprouts, thin slices of cucumber (or thicker slices, if you like the crunch), and turkey slices. Wrap as if it's a burrito, and use toothpicks to close.

CHAPTER TWELVE

Vitamins and Minerals for Prevention and Healing

Most of us do not receive adequate quantities of vitamins and minerals through our foods, and stress or certain lifestyle habits (such as cigarette smoking or excessive alcohol consumption) depletes the vitamin activity within our bodies. Tissues, systems, and organs eventually break down, resulting in an array of illnesses. Food alone isn't concentrated enough to strengthen the weaknesses in tissues and organs, but vitamin and mineral supplementation provide the necessary concentrations for rebuilding the body.

When I first diagnose patients, I usually advise large quantities of vitamins and minerals. However, within three to six months, supplementation is often reduced and, for some people, eliminated altogether within two years.

It's important to note that people who are constantly stressed or who live in polluted cities will always need some supplementation. Those who reside downwind from coal-powered factories or in urban areas such as Los Angeles or New York City require higher concentrations of vitamins C and A to protect the membranes in their respiratory systems than people who live in coastal areas where the air is refreshed by sea breezes. Athletes, construction workers, and others who are physically active require high concentrations of B vitamins, certainly at a level higher than a person who has a desk job.

The following recommendations are for those who are maintaining a proper diet and are under minimal stress. Because physical conditions vary so dramatically among individuals, specific strengths and weaknesses should be determined by a physician familiar with vitamin and mineral therapy.

Type O

Vitamin A: 10,000 IU daily with vitamin D, 800–1,000 mg

Vitamin B: One high-potency stress B-complex tablet per day: 100 mg of B_1, 100 mg of B_2, 100 mg of B_6, 20 mg of B_3, and 500 mg of B_{12}

Pantothenic acid: 250 mg once to twice daily when under stress

Folic acid: 800 mcg daily

Vitamin C: 1,000 mg once or twice daily (more if needed)

Vitamin E: 400 IU daily

Iron: One tablet daily (use homeopathic iron if this causes constipation)

Bone Support: The D'Adamo Institute's formula is two tablets daily, or one to two bonemeal tablets per day

Chelated calcium or calcium gluconate: 500–1,000 mg per day (women generally need 1,000 mg or more)

Multimineral tablet: 1–2 daily

Probiotic: Once or twice a day

Bladder wrack: Take two twice a day

Potassium: 99 mg (1 or 2 tablets)

Type A

Vitamin A: 10,000 IU daily with vitamin D, 800–1000 mg.

Vitamin B: 1–2 low-stress B-complex tablets daily (not made from yeast; made from rice-polished powder): 5–10 mg B_1, 5–10 mg B_2, 10 mg B_3, 100–500 mcg B_{12}, 50 mg B_6

Folic acid: 400 mcg daily

Vitamin C: 250 mg daily (more may be taken if you have a cold; reduce dosage on relief of symptoms)

Vitamin E: 200 IU daily

Hydrochloric acid: 1–3 tablets once a day and ¼ rennet tablet to buffer against acidity; always take chelated calcium with the hydrochloric acid

Calcium gluconate: 500 mg daily for men; 1,000 mg daily for women

Multimineral tablet: 1–2 daily

Digestive enzyme: One tablet taken daily with the heaviest meal

Kelp tablets: 1–2 daily

Potassium: 99 mg (1 tablet per day)

Type B

Vitamin A: 10,000 IU once a day with 800–1,000 mg of vitamin D

Vitamin B: 1–2 medium-potency B-complex tablets every day: 100 mg B_1, 100 mg B_2, 10 mg B_3, and 50 mg B_6; 1–2 100 mg tablets B_{12} daily

Folic acid: 400 mcg daily

Vitamin C: 250 mg twice a day

Vitamin E: 400 IU daily

Multimineral tablet: 1–2 daily

Calcium gluconate or Bone Support: 2–3 tablets daily (about 1,000 mg); or 1–2 bonemeal tablets per day

Iron: One tablet every three days

Type AB

Vitamin A: 10,000 IU daily with 800–1,000 mg of vitamin D

Vitamin B: 1–2 low-potency B-complex tablets every day: 5–10 mg B_1, 5–10 mg B_2, 10 mg B_3, 50 mg B_6, and 100–500 mcg B_{12}

Folic acid: 400 mcg daily

Vitamin C: 250 mg daily

Vitamin E: 200 mg twice a day

Multimineral tablet: 1–2 daily

Calcium gluconate or chelated calcium lactate: 500 mg daily

Hydrochloric acid: 1–2 tablets daily (with ¼ rennet tablet)

Iron: One tablet every ten days

Digestive enzyme: One tablet following a heavy meal

Potassium: 99 mg; one tablet daily

Type Oa

Vitamin A: 10,000 IU once a day with 800–1,000 mg of vitamin D

Vitamin B: One high-potency stress B-complex tablet daily: 100 mg B_1, 100 mg B_2, 20 mg B_3, 100 mg B_6, and 500 mg B_{12}

Folic acid: 800 mcg daily

Pantothenic acid: 250 mg daily

Vitamin C: 1,500 mg daily (more if needed)

Vitamin E: 400 IU daily

Multimineral tablet: 1–2 daily

Calcium chelate: 5 or 6 per day; the best is Bone Support, 3 or 4 tablets per day

Iron: One tablet daily (use homeopathic iron if this causes constipation)

Kelp tablets: 1–3 daily

Type Ob

Vitamin A: 10,000 IU once a day with 800–1,000 mg of vitamin D

Vitamin B: One high-potency stress B-complex daily: 100 mg B_1, 100 mg B_2, 20 mg B_3, 100 mg B_6, and 500 mcg B_{12}

Folic acid: 800 mcg daily

Pantothenic acid: 250 mg (1 to 2 daily when under stress)

Vitamin C: 1,000 mg; 1 to 2 daily (more if needed)

Vitamin E: 400 IU daily

Multimineral tablet: 1–2 daily

Bone support: 2–4 tablets daily

Calcium gluconate: 500–1,000 mg daily (women should take at least 1,000 mg daily)

Bladder-wrack tablets: Take one tablet three times a day or two twice a day

Iron: One tablet daily (use homeopathic iron if this causes constipation)

Potassium: 99 mg; 1 tablet daily

Type Ao

Vitamin A: 10,000 IU once a day with 800–1,000 mg of vitamin D

Vitamin B: 1½ high-stress B tablets every day (one tablet in the morning, ½ tablet in the evening): 100 mg B_1, 100 mg B_2, 20 mg B_3, 100 mg B_6, and 500 mcg B_{12}

Folic acid: 400 mcg daily

Vitamin C: 1,000 mg daily

Vitamin E: 400 IU every day

Multimineral tablet: 1–2 daily

Bone Support: 1–3 daily

Calcium lactate or calcium gluconate: 500 mg daily for men; 1,000 mg for women

Hydrochloric acid: 1–2 tablets once a day (with ¼ rennet tablet to buffer against the acidity) with lunch or dinner

Digestive enzyme: One tablet taken daily with the heaviest meal

Kelp tablets: Two tablets twice a day

Potassium: 99 mg; take one per day

Type Ab

Vitamin A: 10,000 IU once a day with 800–1,000 mg of vitamin D

Vitamin B: Take three low-stress B-complex tablets every day: 5–10 mg B_1, 5–10 mg B_2, 10 mg B_3, 50 mg B_6, and 100–500 mcg B_{12}

Folic acid: 400 mcg daily

Vitamin C: 500–700 mg daily

Vitamin E: 200 IU daily

Multimineral tablet: 1–2 every day

Calcium lactate or calcium gluconate: 500–700 mg daily

Hydrochloric acid: Take one tablet once a day (with ¼ rennet tablet) with lunch or dinner

Kelp tablets: 2–3 daily

Potassium: 99 mg; one per day

Type Bo

Vitamin A: 10,000 IU once a day with 800–1,000 mg of vitamin D

Vitamin B: Two high-stress B-complex tablets every day: 100 mg B_1, 100 mg B_2, 20 mg B_3, 50 mg B_6, and 100–200 mcg B_{12}

Folic acid: 800 mcg daily

Vitamin C: 100 mg twice a day

Vitamin E: 400 IU daily

Multimineral tablet: 1–2 every day

Calcium gluconate or Bone Support: 1,000 mg daily

Iron: One tablet every three days

Potassium: 99 mg; one per day

Type Ba

Vitamin A: 10,000 IU once a day with 800–1,000 mg of vitamin D

Vitamin B: 1–3 low-stress B-complex tablets daily: 5–10 mg B_1, 5–10 mg B_2, 10 mg B_3, 50 mg B_6, and 100–500 mcg B_{12}

Folic acid: 400 mcg daily

Vitamin C: 250 mg daily

Vitamin E: 400 IU daily

Multimineral tablet: 1–2 daily

Calcium gluconate or Bone Support: 500–700 mg daily

Hydrochloric acid: One tablet every day if you are experiencing flatulence; then one tablet every two or three days if you're digesting your food well (always take with ⅛ rennet tablet to buffer against the acidity)

Iron: One tablet every three days

Kelp: 1–2 tablets with meals

Potassium: 99 mg per day or every other day

❧ ❧ ❧

CHAPTER THIRTEEN

Eating Properly

Knowing how to eat can be as important to your health as knowing what to eat. Too few people give this much thought as they file down the health-store aisles squeezing organic tomatoes for ripeness or questioning the fishmonger as to whether the salmon he is filleting was farm raised or caught in the open sea.

As I have said time and again throughout this book, we are in the midst of a wonderful shift as people question the quality and real nutritional value of their foods. But that's only one part of nourishing the body and preventing disease.

There are two equally important aspects to the menus I recommend: The first, of course, is determining *what* foods should be eaten based on a person's blood type and current state of health. The second is knowing *how* these foods should be eaten to promote optimal digestion. Eating properly is often the most challenging part of the diets I create.

I recognize that my recommendations may seem extreme and unreasonable to people, and they often require an entire revolution in a person's eating habits. But the reason patients are in my office with their current conditions is because, for the most part, they have eaten the wrong foods for their individual bodies and are uninformed about the negative effects improper eating habits can have on their health.

I'm sorry to now take the romance or joy out of eating for all of you bons vivants, but once the food that you savor and have given such care to preparing enters the body, it's all about chemistry. That grilled salmon steak is protein with omega-3 fatty acids. Those lovely carrots you passed through an electric juicer are, to me, carotene and sugar. What you may think of as celery, I think of as sodium (one of its major components). The juicy watermelon you bite into on a hot summer's day . . . I see as silica.

Understanding the chemical components of foods helps me determine which foods you should eat to heal your conditions. In order to gain the greatest nutritional value from food, however, you must digest everything to the fullest—which requires interaction with the precise enzymes. No matter how much you eat, undigested or improperly digested meals deprive you of vital vitamins, minerals, and compounds that energize or revitalize your body. I'm sure at some point your mother told you to eat slowly and chew your food well. In today's world, where people multitask or gobble down their meals while clicking a mouse and zooming across the Internet, even less attention or thought is given to proper eating habits than when you sit in front of your TV and eat.

Here's what happens if you don't chew your food well. To start off, you fail to activate your salivary glands to release the needed quantities of ptyalin to be produced. Ptyalin, the enzyme that digests starches, is found in saliva. Starches that are properly chewed move into the stomach with enough ptyalin to digest them in about two hours, but improperly chewed starches may remain in the stomach for up to five hours and even then may not be completely digested.

Proper mastication is only step one in activating the necessary ptyalin. This vital enzyme only works in an alkaline medium, and even mild acids will inhibit its functioning. So if you're eating an acidic food, such as an orange or a pineapple, with a starchy one, such as granola, you're inhibiting proper digestion. But fruits and starches are not the only poor combination. Protein and starch should never be eaten together. The enzyme that initiates protein digestion—pepsin—is produced in the stomach and requires an acid medium in order to work. The ptyalin that initiates the digestion of starches requires an alkaline medium. When both enzymes (pepsin and ptyalin) are secreted together, they neutralize each other. The ptyalin encounters acid and the pepsin encounters alkaline. You can imagine what goes on in your digestive tract when you devour a seemingly innocent roast-beef sandwich or breaded fish and chips.

The following diagram illustrates the way to properly combine foods. As you can see, meat and potatoes, a mainstay of the American diet, is out the window. But vegetables, tofu, nuts, and seeds can be eaten with either animal proteins or starches. Fruits are acid or alkaline in nature, and should be eaten alone.

DO's and DON'Ts and WORDS of ADVICE

1. Never eat when nervous or tense. Even beneficial foods can work adversely under conditions of stress.

2. Never take too hot or too cold foods or liquids. Extreme heat and cold shock the body cells and interfere with the activity of the gastric juices.

3. DO NOT mix a carbohydrate food with an animal protein food during the same meal. The enzymes required to digest carbohydrates differ from those required to digest proteins. If carbohydrates and animal proteins are eaten at the same time, their enzymes neutralize one another, thus minimizing the nutritional value derived from the food. Vegetables are digested within one to one and a half hours; meats and starches take five to eight hours. Follow this food combining guide:

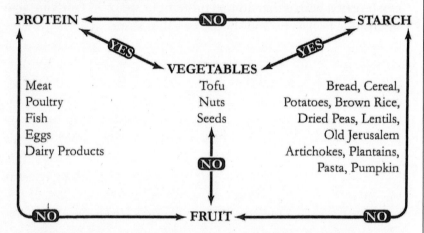

PROTEIN		STARCH
Meat	Tofu	Bread, Cereal,
Poultry	Nuts	Potatoes, Brown Rice,
Fish	Seeds	Dried Peas, Lentils,
Eggs		Old Jerusalem
Dairy Products		Artichokes, Plantains,
		Pasta, Pumpkin

4. Cooking utensils should be made from cast iron, stainless steel, porcelain, enamel or CorningWare. Avoid Teflon, aluminum and plastic utensils.

5. Eat the more laxative foods first; for example, vegetables before meat.

6. Eat foods that are organically cultivated. If they are not available, use fresh or frozen vegetables, never canned. Organic foods are expensive but a wise investment for your future well-being.

7. Eat the vegetables indicated on your menu. Those not indicated should be strictly avoided.

8. All vegetables should be washed thoroughly prior to cooking. Hold vegetables to the light to check for possible insects.

9. Eat at least three to five green vegetables per meal. One quarter package of each frozen vegetable is enough for one meal.

I know the concept of combining food can come as a shock. I've had patients insist that they could never adapt to such a preposterous way of eating! And that not eating turkey, cranberry sauce, and yams at Thanksgiving is un-American! I remind them about how lethargic and bloated they feel after a holiday meal, and that it wasn't only because they ate too much: their digestion was slowed by improper food combining. When proteins are no longer combined with starches, holiday gourmands no longer experience a heaviness in their stomach; they can feel "complete" without having to loosen their belts and open the top button of their trousers.

As you combine your foods properly, digestion will occur more rapidly, and your stomach will feel empty. At first you may experience this change as meaning that you haven't had enough to eat, and you may want a piece of bread or a sweet dessert to fill yourself up. A stomach should be the size of a clenched fist, but improper eating swells it to an unnatural size. This kind of enlargement causes common problems such as hiatal hernias, perforated ulcers, or gastric ulcers. When your stomach shrinks to its normal and healthy size, you'll find that you'll be satisfied by far less food.

Proper combining of food is also one of the primary reasons my patients lose weight naturally. Before treatment, most of my patients' daily menu consists of cereal, toast, and coffee for breakfast; a sandwich and piece of fruit for lunch; and meat, potatoes, and a sweet dessert for dinner. And they often stuff themselves with cookies and doughnuts or other carbohydrates when they're hungry. When you combine food properly, the craving for carbs fades, and those extra pounds drop away effortlessly—and they stay off.

I cannot emphasize enough the importance of eating properly. No longer will your body have to fight against itself to be properly nourished, and this in turn will help your body find its normal energy level.

Ease Into Your New Menu

Before making major changes to your diet, please remember that these require considerable modifications in lifestyle. Most people have been eating poorly all of their lives and are addicted to many foods. It's best to make changes slowly and carefully. For the majority, rigidly adhering to a new menu can be very stressful. Your body is most likely already nutritionally stressed, and you don't want to add to it. Give yourself one to three months to ease into a new menu. Old habits die hard, but once this becomes a way of life, it will seem natural; and you may question how you ever ate any other way.

Shopping

— Look for vegetables that are organically grown. If they aren't available, use fresh or frozen, but never consume canned vegetables. Organic foods are more expensive, but they are a wise investment for your future well-being. Try to find a local organic market, but these days organic food can also be bought at most major supermarkets as well as specialty shops.

— Pick vegetables that are indicated on your menu. Those not listed should be strictly avoided.

— Avoid iceberg lettuce. It contains minimal food value.

— Buy ungassed bananas. Bananas brought to North America from the Caribbean islands are picked unripened and are sprayed with natural ethylene gas for ripening when they arrive. The chemistry of the fruit is altered dramatically.

— Choose fruit juices that are stored in glass containers and contain no added sugar or preservatives.

— Fish should always be fresh. When the eyes of the fish are colorless and gray, it isn't fresh or it has been frozen. There should be a bright red hue behind the gills. Never buy fish that has been filleted or that has had the head removed. Avoid farm-raised fish, as they mature in ponds that are often loaded with fish waste and antibiotics.

— Codfish can be eaten in wintertime from December to April. In the summer, this fish swims closer to the shore and often carries a worm.

— Avoid tuna and swordfish as they contain large quantities of mercury.

— Avoid lobsters, shrimp, and clams because they are scavengers and are more likely to contain higher levels of toxic mercury.

— Much of the meat available at butcher shops is tenderized with steroids. Whenever possible, buy free-range meat that has not been injected.

— Organ meats are far better for the body than muscle meat because they are free of uric acid, which concentrates in muscles.

— When storing tofu, place it in a container with water and keep it covered in the refrigerator. Change the water daily to keep it fresh. Be sure to use it before it becomes slippery, changes color, or tastes sour.

— The harder the cheese, the higher the bacteria count. Softer cheeses, such as mozzarella or ricotta, are preferable.

— Buy fresh nuts. Nuts become rancid quickly.

— With all the delicious, organic alternative milk products available today (such as almond, soy, and rice milk), there is no need to use cow's milk.

— Read all the labels when buying packaged foods. Avoid those containing artificial preservatives either in the food or in the packaging.

Cooking

— Cooking utensils should be made from cast iron, porcelain, enamel, or CorningWare. Avoid Teflon, aluminum, and plastic utensils.

— All vegetables should be washed thoroughly; carefully examine your produce for insects.

— Never boil vegetables; they lose their nutritional value. Vegetables should be eaten raw or steamed. Purchase a steamer insert or a pressure cooker.

— When cooking for extremely ill patients, steam all vegetables; they are more easily digested and passed.

— Check with your doctor before buying a juice-extracting machine, as vegetable juices are highly concentrated foods and may be harmful to you in your current state of health.

— Brown rice should be cooked with two teaspoons of nutritional yeast, which breaks down the rice and makes it more assimilable.

— Dried soybeans should be soaked for 24 hours prior to use. During cooking, the water should be changed each time a white film appears (usually about three times). This will prevent flatulence.

— Never heat or cook natural honey, as heating destroys the enzymes.

— All oils should be fresh and stored in the refrigerator. Grapeseed, flaxseed, or sesame oil is best for cooking. Do not cook with canola oil.

Eating

— Never eat when you're nervous or tense. Even beneficial foods can work adversely if eaten when you're upset or stressed.

— Never drink liquids that are too hot or cold. Extreme heat and cold shock the body's cells and interfere with the activity of the gastric juices and delicate membranes of the esophagus. Be sure to drink plenty of water between meals.

— Eat at least three to five green vegetables per meal.

— Vegetables for breakfast? Yes, if you want to—they're beneficial to eat at any time.

— Do not eat fruits directly before or after a meal. Fruit should be eaten 20 minutes before or 45 minutes after a meal.

— Always wait 30 minutes after drinking vegetable or fruit juices before eating solid food.

— Do not drink during a meal. Water and juice dilute digestive juices.

— Nuts should be chewed thoroughly and should be eaten in small quantities—a handful. Walnuts, almonds, pecans, and sunflower seeds are the most beneficial for you.

— Daily rations of vitamins and supplements should be spaced out and taken with meals. Do not take more than recommended, as too many may be detrimental. Use as little water as possible when taking vitamins, and never take them with juice. Consult with your doctor before taking vitamins or supplements, as they are concentrated food substances. Foods may not be concentrated enough to revitalize your body, so certain vitamins may be prescribed to you for the necessary time period.

— Dried fruits can be eaten by all blood types if they're purchased from a health-food store and if you have no problems with sugar. However, dried fruits are concentrates, so eat small amounts.

Rules

— Do not mix a carbohydrate with a protein food during the same meal. Follow the food combining guide.

— Lunches should generally be vegetarian.

— Do not mix acid and alkaline fruits at the same meal.

— Drink six to eight glasses of water every day. Tap water filtered through a water purifier attached to your sink works well. Also recommended are glass-bottled mineral water and springwater, but strictly avoid carbonated or charged water. Water cleanses the kidneys and kidneys filter the blood. Water will help your kidneys function at peak performance and prevent them from becoming diseased. Never drink water from plastic bottles, as the chemicals in plastic leak into the water. (European bottled waters are particular about describing value and content on the labels, and are preferable. Choose water in green- or blue-tinted glass bottles.)

— Do not eat sugar with a protein; for example, meat followed by a sweet dessert.

— Fasting should be undertaken only after consulting with your health-care provider. Fasting can be shocking to your system. When no food is eaten, the body scavenges food from the colon, which creates fermentation in the system.

— Exercise before eating—not after. Resting after eating allows the blood to circulate to the stomach for proper digestion. Exercise moves blood to the extremities and inhibits digestion.

CHAPTER FOURTEEN

Children's Prevention Program

Promoting health and preventing disease should begin on day one of a person's life. Breast milk is the first nourishment a newborn child should receive, as it contains all the vital nutrients that an infant's body needs . . . and yet right from the beginning, most children are improperly nourished.

No food industry is more standardized in terms of producing foodstuff than the children's food industry, with sugary infant formulas, pureed fruits and vegetables, and creamy cereals. Once children are fed bottled formulas or processed baby food as they get older (such as strained, mashed carrots, bananas, apricots, and so forth), they are, in most cases, starting their young lives off on the wrong track.

Moreover, parents train their kids to eat the way they do—for example, many taste baby food before they give it to their children and, if the taste doesn't suit them, they add salt or sugar. (And most baby foods already contain added salt and sugar to appeal to the parents' taste buds!) Children learn to like what their parents like—so we can expand the maxim "You are what you eat" to "You are what your parents eat, too."

Just like adults, all children should be fed as individuals according to their blood type. By doing so, we can support them so that their bodies and minds will flourish. I've treated children whose parents and grandparents have followed the blood-type diet (my own children and grandchildren have been raised in this manner), and these children clearly experience fewer health problems and also have a more balanced disposition than those who first come to my clinic for guidance or treatment.

All children can be—should be—this healthy and vital. They will develop their innate talents and gifts if their parents monitor their diet and exercise, and use the clues that their children's blood type provides.

Almost 90 percent of children's diseases can be prevented. Most are caused by poor nutritional patterns or emotional upsets. If children are kept away from high-carbohydrate foods and sugar, if their rooms are ventilated at night, if they get adequate exercise and rest, if they are given proper vitamins, if they eat according to blood types, and if they are given emotional security, they will thrive.

Parents also need to remember that the child who has come through them into the world has his or her own mind and destiny. They need to offer guidance with love and positive support, while being conscious of their own habits and actions because their children will emulate them, consciously or otherwise. If you smoke, your children are likely to smoke. If you eat red meat every day and drink a glass of milk with every meal, your children are apt to do the same. If you eat candy when you are upset, your children will follow your example.

Children want to be loved and will do whatever they can to please. And if sickness brings them the attention they crave, they will learn to be sick. Sickness most definitely can be purposely acquired.

Each Child Is Different

John and Edward are brothers. Six-year-old John is thin and wiry with blue eyes and blond hair. Four-year-old Edward is more solidly built, with curly brown hair and dark brown eyes. John is deeply sensitive and very bright; his teachers say he's a brilliant child. Edward is a robust boy who loves to play baseball and ride his bicycle. He claims that he is the toughest boy at the nursery school: "When somebody punches me, I punch them right back and I win." While John spends hours drawing with pencils and paper, Edward prefers to "zoom" his trucks around the playroom.

Although Edward has a tendency to imitate his older brother, it's obvious that over time the two boys will develop radically different interests. John will likely be involved in intellectual and artistic pursuits, while Edward will probably enjoy sports. Even now they have different ambitions. John wants to be an artist, and Edward wants to be a policeman. Dietary preferences are also clear already. John isn't fond of meat, preferring chicken to beef. He loves vegetables and prefers fresh fruit to cookies. Edward, on the other hand, loves hamburgers and peanut butter and hates salads.

These two boys are being raised in the same family, by the same parents, and they sleep in the same room. The food available to them has been the same, and their toys are usually shared. What is different about each child, however, is his blood type. John has Type A blood and Edward has Type O. This difference can alert their parents to their sons' uniqueness and guide them in determining what kind of diet, exercise, and learning environment is best for their children. If these factors are taken into account and acted on appropriately, it is likely that both children can be high achievers at school.

By checking your children's blood types, you can suit their diet and lifestyle to their own particular needs. Obviously, children are not going to be divided into classrooms according to blood type; however, information about what works best for your children when learning can be shared with teachers and can certainly be implemented at home. Adjusting their diets and exercise habits to their blood type can result in academic accomplishments beyond your hopes and dreams for your children.

Finally, here are a few things you can do for your children, regardless of their blood type:

- Make your own baby food with organic vegetables; or if need be, only purchase organic baby food in glass jars.

- Use sippy cups or bottles that are BPA free; plastic bottles can leach a toxic chemical called bisphenol A (BPA) into formula and breast milk.

- And always, always read the ingredients if you're using baby formula instead of breast milk, because many formulas are loaded with chemicals and preservatives. Be mindful of what you feed your child.

The Type-O Child

Type O children must use their bodies. The key to creativity and academic achievement for them is heavy physical exercise. Before class begins and intermittently throughout the day, these children should participate in vigorous physical activity. Games that involve running, such as basketball, are extremely beneficial, for when they are physically active, they become more alert. Such children would do better to run and play before an exam rather than sit quietly and study. These children are "high octane."

Type O students would learn best from teachers who are active and enthusiastic. Teaching methods that involve competition would be effective for these children as they are highly competitive by nature. They would, for example, enjoy spelling bees. Homework assignments would be tackled with gusto for a time; but if the child does not take a break after an hour or so to engage in physical activity, he or she is likely to become bored and tired. Parents should remember that their Type O child requires physical activity.

The rooms in which these children work and play should be decorated in vibrant colors. Bright oranges, yellows, and reds are suitable because these colors resonate with Type O's energy and will support their ability to learn.

Dietary needs include large quantities of protein, usually at two meals per day. Protein is high-energy food, and high energy is what makes Type O children tick.

The Type-A Child

These are the children of the mind, and their energy is that of the nervous system rather than the musculoskeletal system. Type A's love to read and quietly work by themselves. They are good at games that rely on strategy rather than endurance, because their body's energy tends to come through the nervous system.

Type A's are best suited to a serene environment, but if they aren't provided with the type of surroundings that best suit them, these children are likely to be hyperactive and can be mistaken for Type O's. Because their nervous systems are so sensitive, excess stimulation around them creates a frenetic response in the delicate fabric of their bodies. Their nervous systems respond to every sound and movement. These may be the children who are always busy or who are chatterboxes or wigglers. Activity around them creates activity in their bodies. In order for them to use their minds effectively, they must be surrounded by calmness and peace.

Such children would flower with teachers who encourage individual work. They would work with each child individually, offering them understanding and praise. A short walk or a period of yoga or stretching exercises before classes begin would be best for Type A's. Since these children can concentrate for long periods of time if they are properly nurtured, they would not thrive on a curriculum that emphasized a variety of subjects over short periods. Rather, Type A's perform best if they are assigned projects that allow them to use their intellect and creativity. Moreover, competitive games do not appeal to them.

Type A's are best suited to an environment of blues and greens, the calming colors. Because they're more mental than physical, their nutritional needs are unlikely to include large amounts of protein. Lunches should be vegetarian, and dairy products should be eliminated as much as possible. Light foods allow the mind to be quick.

The Type-B Child

These children experience the best of both worlds: they are in between Types O and A. Type B's are natural organizers. They are the kids who get a neighborhood basketball game going. They love to talk and share with others. As a result, they enjoy group activities. They have orderly minds and prefer an uncluttered environment. They are uncomfortable in a classroom where desks are arranged haphazardly, preferring a definite pattern, whether it's rows, circles, or semicircles.

Physically, they also fall in between Types A and O. They benefit from stretching exercises before morning classes and heavy physical exercise before afternoon classes. They are good at team sports. If they take up running, they're most likely to do so with a friend. Type B children like to discuss their homework with their parents, an older sibling, or a friend.

In the classroom, Type B's benefit from group study. They do best with teachers who are leaders and possess excellent communication skills. These teachers would need to be orderly, presenting the child with a well thought-out curriculum. The minds of Type B children operate through relationships; thus, they would want a natural order of subjects throughout the day. History, for example, should follow geography rather than mathematics.

Because of their innate flexibility, Type B's are comfortable with the full spectrum of color. Whether their room is yellow, orange, blue, or green, these children will be able to function well.

Lunches for these children should be balanced between high protein and lighter foods. Only one meal a day should contain protein.

The Type-AB Child

These children may carry traits of both Type A's and Type B's, in varying quantities. To understand the Type AB child, parents should read the sections on both of these blood groups. These children usually have a delicate nervous system and are often intellectual by nature. They are usually very creative, and this may surface in the social activities they participate in, such as theater or gymnastics.

To determine whether the A or the B is dominant, parents should examine their children carefully. Should they suffer from mucous conditions, have a great deal of nervous energy, and experience difficulty concentrating, then they probably lean toward the A type. Recommendations for Type A's would probably be helpful here. On the other hand, if children enjoy spending time with friends, love organizing and mediating, and excel at strategizing in sports, then they probably lean toward the B type. Recommendations for Type B's may be helpful here.

Type AB's benefit most from stretching or yoga, yet some may require heavy physical activity. Their teachers need to be alert to the ways in which their creativity and intellect are best nurtured. Some Type AB students may prefer to work alone on projects while others prefer to work in groups.

Their diet should lean toward lighter foods with few animal proteins and a minimum of dairy products.

Family Menus

It isn't always easy to watch what our children eat. They have minds of their own, and as they get older, they will experiment and be attracted to new cultures and foods.

All this is complicated by the fact that there can be individuals in the family with different blood types. Where do you begin? As I've said throughout this book, get rid of the sugars, candies, junk food, and processed foods. These are not good for anyone. Add more green vegetables, which everyone needs.

Plan menus around those items that are good for all blood types in your family. Start with a basic that everyone can eat, and then add a little meat here for the Type O individual, and reduce eggs there for the Type A. Do the best you can.

And keep in mind that children imitate their parents. Remember the Type A boy who suffered with asthma? Although his condition improved quickly after his parents eliminated dairy products, his symptoms roared back when he ate sweets with his father after dinner.

Doing what is best for our children is not always easy, but it pays off in the long run by protecting their health and vitality.

CHAPTER FIFTEEN

Children's Illnesses and Remedies

It is inevitable that children will develop an illness or physical condition as they grow. Some conditions, such as teething, are painful to endure but part of the maturing process; and illnesses, such as the measles, help children build immunity and actually strengthen their system as they grow into adulthood. Whether illnesses or growing pains, these experiences can be stressful for both children and parents.

This chapter contains possible causes and treatments for common childhood conditions. The heart of my belief and this program as I've described throughout this book is proper diet according to blood type. My children and grandchildren have all been nourished according to their type of blood and have had exceptionally healthy and vital lives.

At times, however, conditions such as diaper rash, ear infection, or childhood eczema may require additional therapies, including herbal preparations or homeopathic remedies to promote the healing process. I've made a variety of such recommendations where appropriate.

Hopefully, this list will broaden your understanding of your child's condition and help you respond more calmly and confidently to his or her needs. As always, my suggestions should be made in consultation with your physician.

Asthma

Possible causes: The incidence of asthma has escalated in the past decade, particularly among children in urban areas; and air pollution is one of the primary causes of this condition. Airways become sensitized and inflamed, and further exposure to irritants in the air—and chemicals in the household—can exacerbate and trigger this disease.

Treatment: Asthma is also a condition that tells us that waste products are not being eliminated properly through the kidneys and bowels. It is essential that asthmatic children are regularly eliminating wastes from the body and that their kidneys are being flushed with water. They must drink large quantities of water, preferably eight to ten glasses daily, to cleanse the bowels and thin the mucus in the respiratory system. If a child refuses to drink a lot of water, fruit juice may be substituted, but it should be diluted with water.

Regardless of blood type, all dairy products should be removed from the diet, as should all sweets, including cakes, chocolate, ice cream, and cookies. Meat consumption should also be reduced. Substitute soy milk for whole milk and avoid cheese. In addition, children should eat lots of green vegetables and take extra vitamin A, D, and C to strengthen their immune system.

All dry heat and central heating must be shut off; windows should be opened to provide proper ventilation. I recommend that children suffering from asthma should sleep with their head elevated three to four inches higher than their feet to promote easier breathing.

A mixture containing two ounces of a tincture of Grindelia, 20 drops of osha, plus 15 drops of a tincture of echinacea and vitamin C is effective in treating acute asthma. Use 10 drops in a teaspoon of lukewarm water, three to five times a day.

There are also many homeopathic remedies for asthmatic conditions, but these must be used in consultation with a qualified physician. They include ferrum phosphoricum dose potency 30C (two tablets, two times a day) or silica 30C (two tablets, two times a day as needed).

Other homeopathic options and the situations in which you should use them are as follows:

- Aconite 30C: Asthmatic symptoms come on suddenly (often in extreme in winter); onset often follows a shock or chill to cold weather.

- Phosphorous 30C: Asthmatic children desire ice-cold drinks, are very thirsty, and/or experience bright red nosebleeds. Breathing improves when placed in a sitting position with neck and head arched back.

- Kali carbonicum 30C: Use when symptoms appear to worsen (oftentimes between 2 and 4 A.M.); coughing may decrease after vomiting.

- Antimonium tartaricum 30C: You hear a rattle sound in the chest, but it's too difficult for the child to cough up mucus; symptoms are worse in a warm room and appear to decrease when in open air and sitting up.

Colic

Possible causes: This is a digestive complaint brought on by improper diet or wrong food combination, and the excessive production of air in a child's digestive tract. Eliminate refined sugar and carbohydrates. Parents should remember that certain vegetables (like sweet potatoes) are loaded with sugar and to limit these as well.

Treatment: Follow the child's diet for his or her blood type, and add probiotics and B complex. Homeopathic options and the situations in which you should use them include:

- Colocynthis 30C: This is a typical remedy for colic. Children typically feel better when they are bending forward.

- Magnesium phosphoricum 30C: Pain is better with heat and gentle pressure applied on belly.

- Chamomile 30C: The child is irritable and wants to be carried, not cuddled. The child is always thirsty and has green, foul-smelling stool.

- Lycopodium 30C: Symptoms are worse between 4 and 8 P.M. The child craves sweets; throat feels better with warm drinks.

Common Cold

Possible causes: One of the main reasons children get colds is because their rooms are not properly ventilated, which often results in headaches and head colds. The combination of dry air and increased carbon dioxide over the night creates the perfect environment for colds. Another contributing factor is the ingestion of large quantities of junk food and excess dairy products. These foods increase quantities of mucus in the body and clog the bowels.

Treatment: Bedroom windows and doors should be left open at night. A humidifier in the room is also helpful. In addition, all blood types should be given increased quantities of vitamin C (preferably with echinacea) and vitamin A. If the cold is in the bronchial tree, take the child into the bathroom and turn on the hot water to create steam, which will assist breathing. A vaporizer with eucalyptus oil added can also help. The head of the bed should be raised four to five inches as well. It's important for the child to drink a lot of fluids to promote bowel movements.

If the child is coughing but has no phlegm, use a mustard plaster: Mix 100g of flour with two tablespoons of dried mustard.

Spoon a hole in the center of the mixture, and stir in enough hot water to make a paste. Then spread the paste on a cotton dish towel and apply it to the child's chest, paste-side up—that is, the clean cloth, *not* the side with the paste, should rest on the child's skin to prevent a burn. The child should remain lying down until the heat of the plaster can be felt (about three to four minutes). Then the child should flip over, and the plaster can be applied to the back for another three to four minutes. An adult should stay with the child throughout this process. Never use a plaster on an infant.

Following the removal of the plaster, give the child a cup of strong rose-hip tea with one tablespoon of honey and one teaspoon of brandy. The child should remain in bed and under the sheets; sweating may occur and pajamas and bedclothes may need to be changed. Vitamin C should also be taken every two hours throughout the day.

Homeopathic options and the situations in which you should use them include:

- Ferrum phosphoricum 30C: Use during the first stage of a cold, especially if the cold came on slowly, and the child has a low fever.

- Gelsemium 12C: Administer if the child is drowsy, has droopy eyes, and his or her limbs feel heavy.

- Pulsatilla 30C: If the child feels better in open air, and thick yellow discharge is expelled from nose; the child is weepy and needy.

Diaper Rash

Possible cause: This is most often caused by chafing of the skin by damp or soiled disposable diapers or even cotton diapers.

Treatment: Make a salve of 5 tablespoons of calendula ointment, 1 to 2 capsules of vitamin E, a drop or two of cod-liver oil, and a dab of zinc oxide. Applying the blended salve after each diaper change will help reduce mild irritations and rashes. I also recommend adding baking soda to a warm bath. Bathe the child for 15 to 20 minutes to help dry out the rash.

Homeopathic options and the situations in which you should use them include:

- Sulfur 30C: The child has patches of red, itchy skin that are made worse by warmth and bathing.

- Rhus toxicodendron 30C: The child's skin is worse when wet and cold, and is particularly worse at night. The child is restless, and symptoms appear to decrease with heat and movement.

Diarrhea

Possible cause: Improper food combining and excessive consumption of carbohydrates can cause diarrhea.

Treatment: Increase B complex and add acidophilus to the diet. A baked sweet potato, brown rice, cooked green vegetables, and rye bread will help bind the stomach and reduce or relieve the symptoms.

Homeopathic options and the situations in which you should use them include:

- Podophyllum 30C: Urgent morning diarrhea (pea soup–like) and colic; gets worse between 4 and 5 A.M.; very gassy; very weak.

- Nux vomica 30C: For nausea or vomiting due to over-eating. Extremely irritable and sensitive to noise.

- Arsenicum album 30C: The diarrhea is relieved with warm applications applied on belly. Use when diarrhea increases after cold foods and drinks, especially after eating ice cream.

Ear Infection

Possible causes: The most common cause of an ear infection is improper diet, which can result in a postnasal drip that produces an infection in the ears, nose, or throat.

Treatment: Dairy products should be eliminated (regardless of blood type) until the symptoms have passed. If the problem is recurrent, dairy products should be reduced permanently. Add acidophilus to diet. Apply Citricidal ear drops (a combination of grapefruit and tea-tree oil) in the ear.

Ear drops of a mullein solution are also effective in reducing infections. Inhaling a blend of water and eucalyptus oil from a vaporizer can help reduce inflammation.

Homeopathic options and the situations in which you should use them include:

- Belladonna 30C: Use when ear infection comes on suddenly with high fever. Check extremities: if they are cold but the head feels hot, this is a good homeopathic to use.

- Chamomile 30C: The child is irritable and wants to be carried, not cuddled. Green and foul-smelling stool.

Eczema

Possible causes: Eczema may be caused by faulty elimination of the bowels. If there is poor elimination and toxins cannot be eliminated through the kidneys, then the next organ available to aid in elimination is the skin.

Treatment: To reverse such conditions, the child's body must be cleansed and the appropriate blood-type diet must be adhered to. Eliminate dairy and wheat. Type O's should temporarily stop eating dairy and flesh foods, but after the body is cleansed, they can be reintroduced. Type A's should stay away from all dairy and flesh food permanently. Vitamins A and E are especially important.

Homeopathic remedies can include Rhus toxicodendron 30C (two tablets, two times a day) or homeopathic sulfur 30C (two tablets, two times a day).

Oatmeal baths are soothing to a child's inflamed skin. Wrap a handful of oatmeal in a handkerchief and immerse in a bath of warm water. A 15-minute soak will relieve itching and coat the child's skin with a healing, creamy milk.

Fever

Fevers of 100 to 102 degrees should not be considered dangerous in children. The raised temperature simply indicates that the body's immune system is rallying. When a child has an infection, the hypothalamus produces a fever to allow the blood to circulate faster, bringing antibodies and white blood cells to the affected areas in order to envelop the bacteria. When we give our children aspirin to combat a fever, we slow down the flow of blood, and the antibodies cannot reach affected areas quickly. Bacteria are thus enabled to spread at an increased rate. It is important to recognize that low-grade fevers can be helpful to children.

Possible cause: Fevers that are not accompanied by other symptoms are probably related to the ingestion of junk food. Carbohydrates and sugary foods produce large amounts of morbid material in the digestive system. Until this has been excreted, the child may have a fever.

Treatment: With correct supervision from a professional, one or two enemas may be enough to reduce the fever. I cannot over-emphasize the importance of cleaning the bowels. In addition, the child should be given plenty of liquid; the body must not be allowed to dehydrate. Homeopathic ferrum phosphoricum 6X under the tongue can be helpful. Vitamin C and echinacea can be given for cold and flu symptoms. Goldenseal tea, chamomile tea, or homeopathic nux vomica may also provide relief for stomach distress.

Additional homeopathic options and the situations in which you should use them include:

- Belladonna 30C: Use when ear infection comes on suddenly with high fever; check extremities—if they are cold but the head feels hot, this is an effective treatment.

- Gelsemium 30C: Use if the child is drowsy, has droopy eyes, and his or her limbs feel heavy.

Sore Throat

Possible causes: Children frequently suffer from sore throats and sinus trouble. Common causes are improper eating and/or elimination, as well as postnasal drip and tonsillitis.

Treatment: Grate a raw carrot and place the grated carrot in a cotton cloth. Fold the cloth over and wrap around the throat for 15 to 20 minutes twice a day. An alternative is to prepare a cabbage poultice in the same way you would prepare a carrot poultice. In addition, a solution of tepid water and ¼ teaspoon of salt or a solution of two-thirds water and one-third vinegar can be gargled. Vitamins C and A should be taken every two hours. Use Citricidal drops for sore throats.

Stomachache

Possible causes: Stomachaches are often due to improper elimination of the bowels, tension, and the wrong combination of foods.

Treatment: It is often difficult for parents to imagine that tension could enter their child's world. Children do not need to make mortgage payments and do not have concerns about a career. However, they do participate in a society of other children, and what looks like a minor disappointment to a parent can feel like a major catastrophe to a child. Such upsets can affect the digestive system. Oftentimes, a stomachache will go away if a parent or caregiver spends some quiet time with the child and talks about the upsetting incident.

Parents should also check on the foods the child has been eating. If a lot of sweets have been consumed or new foods have been added to the diet, the child may feel ill. Do not let the child eat anything for a while, but do provide frequent, small quantities of water. Goldenseal tea is very helpful, one tablespoon at a time. Always treat stomach conditions with bitters, not sweets. Slippery-elm and dandelion teas are also effective treatments.

If the child has not moved his or her bowels for a few days, this could result in a stomachache. An enema may be the treatment of choice; however, never give a child who has a stomachache an enema until a qualified physician has ruled out appendicitis.

Finally, if the stomachache persists for more than one day, your child should be examined by a physician.

Homeopathic remedies and the situations in which you should use them include:

- Nux vomica 12C or 30C: Used to soothe a wide variety of stomach disorders, including nausea and digestive allergic reactions.

- Chamomilla 30C: This is excellent for colic and stomachaches caused by sluggish or constipated bowels.

Teething

Teeth begin developing while your baby is in the womb, as tooth buds form in the gums. Teeth break through one at a time over a period of months and years and can cause much discomfort. Symptoms to watch for are gum swelling and sensitivity and irritability or fussiness, along with sleep problems (for both baby and parent!).

Treatment: Dip a clean washcloth in a tea of chamomile, elderberry, peppermint, and echinacea. Freeze the soaked cloth, and allow the child to chew on it. This helps reduce inflammation and prevent infection. Adding a few drops of clove oil will also help in decreasing pain.

A homeopathic option to use is chamomile 12C or 30C or teething pellets.

Tonsillitis

Possible cause: Tonsillitis is an inflammation of the lymph nodes in the back of the throat and is generally caused by bacteria or allergies. Inflamed tonsils swell up, turn red, and develop a filmy coat; swallowing becomes painful.

Many years ago, inflamed tonsils were automatically removed. It was believed that they had no value; however, we now know that they are the protectors of the sinus and the throat because they help prevent infection. Parents should do everything possible to avoid surgery. Seek the advice of a physician whose leanings are toward natural therapies.

Treatment: Regardless of blood type, all dairy products should be reduced. Increase intake of vitamin C, especially vitamin C with echinacea. Carrot and cabbage poultices and mists containing tea-tree oil can also be helpful. There are a number of homeopathic remedies for tonsillitis, but I recommend that you consult a qualified physician and not self-medicate.

CHAPTER SIXTEEN

Self-Help Therapies for Common Conditions

I repeat what I wrote at the beginning of this book: I believe that differences in health needs according to blood type is a Truth of nature and that following your individual plan can help heal serious diseases, such as hypoglycemia and cancer, and also help prevent diseases and the misery they cause. Proper care of the body will support the immune system, guard against illness, and provide individuals with long, healthy lives.

Every patient I've treated has heard me say again and again that I've never healed anyone. Nature is the healer. Nature gives us what it wants in terms of healing and strength as soon as we provide the environment and support for it to do its work.

I also firmly believe that no one is alive by mistake and that everyone has a purpose, a destiny, if you will. Where I differ from many who hold the same spiritual concept is that I believe that you can only meet that destiny when you feed your body the way it is meant to be nourished. This allows your body and mind to work in unison so that your spirit can realize its goal on Earth. When body, mind, and spirit are in sync, functioning to the height of their abilities, then many of the conditions and diseases that compromise a person's well-being and enjoyment of life can be prevented.

The path to optimal health and the realization of your life's work, however, is not necessarily a smooth one, and it's not unusual to encounter bumps and detours along the way. In this chapter, I've provided suggestions that you can use to treat some basic ailments (remembering, of course, that you should consult your physician if your ailments persist or worsen). Also remember that more serious conditions may develop if you do not attend to your current conditions in a timely fashion; and finally, never attempt self-healing of a chronic, degenerative disease.

Acid Stomach

Causes: Stomach acidity may result from poor food combining, eating foods that are inappropriate for your blood type, eating too fast, and stress.

Treatment: Probiotics and charcoal tablets are effective in neutralizing stomach acidity. Sprinkling turmeric on your vegetables will also help alleviate an acid stomach.

Acne

Causes: Acne may be caused by excessive consumption of fried foods, sweets, chocolate, candies, and dairy products; as well as poor elimination of the bowels, stress, excessive oil in the skin, hormonal changes with puberty, and air pollution (it isn't uncommon for city dwellers to move to the country and find that their skin clears up).

Treatments: Increase vegetables and roughage in the menu. Type O's should increase intake of whole wheat and grains. Type A's should increase green vegetables. Dairy foods should be decreased. Fried foods and shellfish should be eliminated, as well as sweets, including soda, sugary beverages, and chocolate. Vitamin A can be increased.

Moreover, deodorant soaps should be eliminated. Instead, cleanse the face three times a day with glycerine soap, alternating warm and cold water. If skin is oily, add a pinch of salt to the water, pat onto the skin, and allow to air dry. (This can cause the skin to dry and result in scaling; do not be concerned about this as it's simply old skin coming off.) If there are scars on the skin, apply vitamin E ointment or aloe-vera ointment.

Hair should be washed daily. Individuals with acne should engage in a lot of outdoor exercise—at least one hour per day. If bowel movements don't occur daily, add bran, psyllium seeds, or flaxseed oil to cereal in the morning. Drink at least eight glasses of water a day.

Athlete's Foot

Cause: This condition generally appears in the summer and is caused by a fungus.

Treatment: The best treatment is to expose your feet to the air. Make sure you dry your feet thoroughly after a shower and wear sandals. Athlete's foot develops when damp feet are covered by socks and shoes, which creates the environment for the fungus to grow. Tea-tree oil is also effective for treating the fungus.

Bad Breath

Cause: Bad breath is often due to poor digestion and elimination.

Treatment: It is imperative that you eliminate fast foods and greatly reduce carbohydrates. Combine foods properly, and drink eight glasses of water a day. Colonic irrigation can help improve your elimination system.

Chemical Sensitivities

Cause: The increased use of chemicals in the home and work environment has produced numerous conditions, including allergies, headaches, and chronic nausea. For example, paint, carpeting, chemical cleansers, wood paneling made of formaldehyde, drywall from China, and asbestos have brought a new man-made kind of toxicity into our lives.

Treatment: Be mindful of your household cleaning products. Eliminate as many as you can, and use only those that are biodegradable. An ionizer can help purify the air. And of course, you should try to eat foods that are not grown with chemicals and pesticides.

Colds

Causes: Colds and flu generally tell us that we have pushed our bodies, and our immune systems have been taxed by stress, exposure to cold and dampness, or an excessive amount of work.

Treatment: Increase intake of vitamins C, A, and D. Double intake of B complex, zinc, and magnesium. Be sure to drink plenty of fluids and warm drinks. If the cold is accompanied by a sore throat, gargle with salt water or tea-tree oil (½ teaspoon of either in tepid water) two to three times a day. Echinacea is also excellent for colds, and osha can be taken for chest congestion.

Constipation

Causes: Constipation may be caused by stress, improper diet, wrong food combining, insufficient exercise, or a reliance on pain relievers and medications that interfere with proper digestion.

Treatment: Eliminate medications (in consultation with your physician), drink eight glasses of water a day, increase leafy green vegetables, reduce meats and carbohydrates, increase olive oil, and take a teaspoon or two of flaxseed oil per day.

Diarrhea

Causes: This condition is often caused by tainted foods, improper food combining, stress, and anxiety.

Treatment: Eliminate all processed and junk foods. A combination of cooked white rice, baked sweet potato, and rye bread will bind the stomach and tighten up the bowels. If food poisoning is present, take nux vomica (30C) three times a day.

Flatulence (Gas)

Causes: Bloating is often due to bad food combining or rancid foods. Talking while eating and swallowing air will also produce gas.

Treatment: Add probiotics for three meals, and sprinkle turmeric powder on your vegetables to help eliminate gas. Avoid carbonated drinks.

Headache

Causes: Headaches are often due to misalignment of cervical vertebrae, stress, irregular menstrual flow, and improper food combining.

Treatment: Increase intake of water and olive and flaxseed oils to improve elimination. Add B complex, vitamin C, iron, and desiccated liver. Once the headache abates, increase exercise according to blood type. Chiropractic treatments can realign the vertebrae; acupuncture is also excellent for pain abatement.

Heavy-Metal Toxicity

Cause: This is attributed to chemicals in food and the environment. Symptoms are wide-ranging and can include skin and respiratory allergies, dizziness, fatigue, autoimmune conditions, and arthritis.

Treatment: Blend the following in a juice extractor:

5 celery stalks
5 romaine lettuce leaves
8 pieces of Italian parsley (including stems)
5 pieces of coriander (leaves and stems)
2 Tbsp. soy or rice milk
½ Tbsp. organic honey
½ courgette or squash

If you have been diagnosed with heavy-metal toxicity, I recommend that you drink one glass of this juice three to five times a week.

Jet Lag

Cause: Jet lag is often due to long-distance travel and lack of exercise during a flight.

Treatment: Take melatonin before a long flight and the first night after a flight. Increase water intake and refrain from eating airline food. Wearing an ionizer on a chain will improve the quality of recycled air you breathe during a long flight.

Leg Cramps

Cause: Chronic leg cramps can indicate plaque in the arteries and occlusion of vessels in the legs. This should be checked out medically.

Treatment: Adhering to a diet according to your blood type, increasing magnesium and zinc, and taking daily walks can help reduce acute leg cramps.

Lower-Back Pain

Causes: Overextension of the body, misalignment of vertabrae, constipation, and hormonal imbalance can affect alignment.

Treatment: Reduce dairy and meat intake while treating back pain. Increase calcium and vitamin C. Arnica rubs or moist compresses applied to the lower back can be relieving. Chiropractic treatment, acupuncture, swimming, and light yoga to elongate the back muscles may also provide relief of this common condition.

Menstrual Cramps

Causes: Menstrual cramps are often caused by hormonal imbalance or poor diet with an excessive amount of carbohydrates and sugar.

Treatment: Decrease carbohydrates and eliminate sugar from your daily diet. Blend tinctures of black cohosh, dong quai, and Hypericum in equal parts (10 to 15 drops each). Take 30 drops three to four times a day, five days a week.

Poor Sleep

Causes: Interrupted sleep is different from insomnia and is generally caused by stress and an overactive and troubled mind.

Treatment: Processing and thinking through the problems encountered during the day can help improve the quality of your sleep. If you are under stress and waking up at night, do not get up and leave your bed. Try to quiet your mind and relax your body by doing breathing exercises and meditating. You will drift off to sleep, even though they may be only short bursts of sleep. Much of the time you won't even realize that you've fallen asleep.

Take melatonin (3 to 5 mg) an hour or so before you go to bed. Do not take it right before sleep so that it doesn't interfere with the release of your natural melatonin. Tincture of valerian or Passiflora (15 to 20 drops before going to bed) can also be effective in relaxing the mind and promoting sleep.

Tooth Care

Causes: Teeth can act as a mirror of your nutrition and general health. Tooth decay and many toothaches are often caused by excessive intake of sugar and carbohydrates, smoking cigarettes, and poor dental hygiene.

Treatment: Many people live under the misconception that smoking cigarettes is only bad for your lungs, but it is very damaging to your gums. In addition, failing to floss regularly will cause bleeding and receding gums, which will lead to tooth loss.

Brush your teeth after meals and floss at least before going to bed. Also be mindful of your choice of toothpaste. Many commercial brands contain fluoride and other chemicals that can be detrimental to your health. Tea-tree oil toothpaste is especially good for your teeth and gums and can be purchased at a health-food store.

Here's a recipe for making homemade toothpaste:

½ tsp. baking soda
½ tsp. green clay (the French export an excellent clay; available at health-food stores)
1–2 Tbsp. soy milk
2 drops of ginger

Mix and refrigerate. This is good for about six brushings.

Amalgam fillings contain mercury, which can migrate into the body and cause many conditions. Dentists are increasingly aware of this and are using safer substances; talk to your dentist if you have any old fillings. In addition, increase calcium and vitamins C, A, and D.

Vomiting and Nausea

Causes: Vomiting and nausea generally result from eating bad-quality foods. Excessive eating, eating too rapidly, or even drinking while eating can also induce nausea.

Treatment: Ginger (food or tea) or Liquorice can settle the stomach. Liquorice tablets between meals and sucking on a liquorice stick will calm the condition.

AFTERWORD

I fully believe that the human experience has meaning and purpose, and that each one of us has a realizable destiny. But to aspire to and fulfill that destiny, we must possess mental clarity and physical well-being.

Nature is very generous with each of us. Most people are given physical, emotional, and spiritual health when they are born. We are prepared for our journey into life. How we care for ourselves, our children, our neighbors, and our environment largely determines the quality of our lives and future success and fulfillment.

But can food *really* be the source of your success or failure in life? It would seem like an absurd hypothesis. However, proper nutrition, especially according to your blood type, is at the root of how well you prosper. Eating and exercising in accordance with what nature has provided and intended for your body and your being is key to maximizing your strength, mental acuity, spiritual acumen, and subsequently, your destiny.

My work over the years has helped many people prevent disease and others recover their health. Equally as important, it has helped many find the path that fate has set for them. But I don't take credit for that. I know through years of research and experimentation that nature has provided us with the road map to a healthy, fulfilled life. All I do is encourage people to stay true to themselves—their unique and individual makeup as defined by their blood.

I hope you've read this book in the spirit in which it was written, and that it helps lead you to vibrant health and greater fulfillment.

Diagnostic Procedures

When examining a patient, I use three tools: pulse diagnosis, blood typing, and iridology. Diagnosis is actually an interplay between these three methods. By taking the pulse first, I get a general idea of possible weaknesses. Blood typing usually affirms my findings and allows me to focus my attention on particular factors. Finally, iridology validates the other two. I then can come to concrete decisions about what produces symptoms and what specific menu, exercise plan, supplements, and therapies will reverse known conditions. Since I've discussed blood typing at length, here are brief explanations on iridology and pulse diagnosis.

Signs in the Eyes: Iridology

By examining my patients' irises, I'm able to see all of the weaknesses they have produced in their bodies since birth. It's as if the iris were the recorder for the body. In the following diagram, the landmarks are identified.

Patient Name: _____ **Blood Type:** _____ **Date of Exam:** _____

D'ADAMO IRIS ANALYSIS

Normal Levels

Mucous 0 ——— 4+

Toxicity 0 ——— 5

Total 0 ——— 9

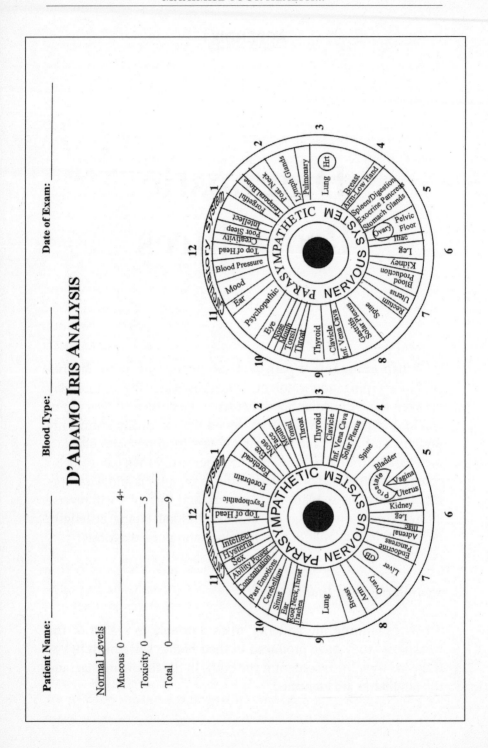

Each landmark corresponds with specific areas of the body. The eye is zonal: the 12 o'clock position represents one area (the head), while another position, say 6 o'clock, represents another (the leg). By holding a mirror close to your eye and then shining a flashlight onto the mirror, you will see various markings on the iris. There may be black spots or white circles, for instance; and each indicates various weaknesses in the body.

The first inner circle represents the sympathetic and parasympathetic nervous systems. Jutting out from the circle may be stress lines. If they are fine speckles, the individual has a tendency to hold stress within the body; that is, the temper is never let out. If the speckling is placed inside the circle as well as on the rest of the iris, the individual releases tension through temper tantrums.

There are other circles in the eyes that I refer to as rings of toxicity. Zero is perfection while five is the highest level possible. One in 800 people will have five rings of toxicity. However, these can be reduced as eating habits are improved and as colon irrigations are taken. As the rings disappear, fewer and fewer colon irrigations are needed.

Mucous clots are little, round, yellowish or whitish clumps on the retina close to the circulatory-system ring. Sometimes they are so severe they reach the nervous system. This signifies that individuals have overburdened their bodies with dairy products. If such spots are seen, dairy products should be eliminated from the diet regardless of blood type until the condition is removed. If this warning is ignored, high blood pressure, clogged arteries, frequent colds, cold feet, cold hands, dizziness, or lapses in memory may occur.

Acute conditions in the body appear as a whiteness with a little yellow. If such a mark appears, for example, in the area identified as sinuses, the individual probably has daily sinus attacks. As treatment progresses, the white turns to gray, and the condition is no longer acute. Eventually, it will become black as the condition leaves, and the iris will return to its original color.

If there is a dark elliptical mark on the iris, there has been a condition in the past that was resolved. If the outside of the mark has white superimposed over it, the condition has once again become acute. Genetic conditions also appear as dark spots and will take some time to resolve. If people have problems with the adrenals, they may be under great strain or have arthritis. If they also show a weakness in the pancreas, then they probably have diabetes. In addition, a mark in the liver area may mean that at one time an individual was taking large doses of medication. If this intake of drugs went on for a very long time, it's possible that the spleen will show a weakness. However, a splenic weakness may mean that an individual contracted mononucleosis at one time. Lung plus kidney weakness usually indicates asthma.

Pulse Diagnosis

When I talk about the pulses, I don't mean the orthodox pulse used by medical doctors or even the Asian pulse. I've developed my own system as a diagnostic tool. (The pulse is taken with three fingers; the thumb should be on the back of the wrist.)

The following is a brief description of what each pulse means. However, this is not intended for self-diagnosis, as "reading" the pulse requires training and clinical practice. It is rather complicated and takes many months to learn. (Physicians or practitioners who are interested in learning my method of pulse diagnosis can contact my institute to arrange training sessions.)

Each area is checked by a finger. If the finger that lies over the pulse feels a feeble beat compared with the others, that may indicate fatigue. If it's really feeble, exhaustion is probably present. Blood may also be circulating poorly.

With the middle pulse, if the beat is high, the acid level is probably high. If it's low, the acid level is probably low. It is likely that an A blood type will have hypoacidity, and an O blood type will have hyperacidity.

With the last pulse, a slow, sluggish beat indicates poor evacuation of the bowels and probably constipation. A very strong pulse signifies diarrhea or colitis. On some occasions, however, a low thready pulse will indicate colitis.

On the left side, the finger that tests the kidney pulse may find a weak beat. This indicates improper fluid intake or a possible kidney or bladder problem.

The middle pulse reflects the functioning of the small intestine. If there is a low pulse, food is fermenting in the small intestine. If the pulse is high, the individual tends not to chew his or her food properly. This person probably gulps food down. If the pulse is thready, the food isn't broken down properly.

The last pulse measures the gallbladder and liver, and reveals how well bile is emulsifying fats. If the pulse is very high, the gallbladder is under strain.

Treatments of the D'Adamo Institute

The following are a variety of treatments used at the D'Adamo Institute.

Herbs, Vitamins, and Supplements

Over years of research, the D'Adamo Institute has developed vitamin supplements formulated for each blood type. In addition, individuals are prescribed single-unit vitamins in order to receive a customized and controlled supplementation. The body receives exactly what it needs at a particular time and—just as important—does not receive what it doesn't need.

Individual requirements and tolerances guide recommendations of herbs and vitamins for every patient. As a patient's health improves, supplements are gradually decreased until eventually a minimal amount or none at all are required.

Inhalation

Our specially designed inhalation apparatus, imported from Germany, allows for the inhalation of various vapors to affect the sinuses and lungs. The herbal tinctures producing these vapors are custom blended in Germany for the D'Adamo Institute.

Water Therapies

Colon Irrigation

Our colon irrigation system eliminates wastes and poisons from the body. Therapies are given in immaculately clean surroundings. The institute follows strict hygienic principles, and equipment is scrupulously maintained. Sterilization by autoclave destroys all germs and viruses.

Constitutional Hydrotherapy

The alternate application of hot and cold wet packs, along with mild electronic stimulation, is used to balance the circulatory and nervous systems. This therapy promotes cell oxygenation, the elimination of toxins, and the proper functioning of the body's defenses.

German Footbath

Used extensively by health spas throughout Europe, footbaths with special herbs are an excellent means of eliminating waste and toxins from the circulatory system.

Physical Therapy Immersion Bath

Our skin is the body's largest organ as well as the most exposed and accessible. Immersion in water enriched with detoxifying herbs allows the skin to become a major exit point for built-up poisons in the body.

At the same time, skin can absorb healing herbs through opened pores. With the addition of special herbal preparations— carefully selected for their healing ability—the therapy tank provides an effective immersion bath treatment. This multifaceted therapy unit functions as an effective treatment for repair of muscular strains, lower-back problems, and shoulder and arm pain, as well as arthritic conditions and the overall relaxation of the nervous system.

This therapy works particularly well when administered in conjunction with a clay-pack or fango treatment application, helping to intensify and deepen the detoxifying effect.

Touch Therapies

Acupuncture

Our staff utilizes auricular, electric, and traditional forms of acupuncture, incorporating techniques practiced for more than 5,000 years.

Aromatherapy

Essential oils extracted from various aromatic plants and trees are utilized for their specific effects on particular organs. During a light massage, these oils produce a cleansing effect in the body's lymphatic system.

Cranial Manipulation

The old concept of the skull as one immovable bone has been revised with the newer scientific understanding that the plates of the skull actually expand and contract rhythmically eight times per minute. When the sutures become fixed, it can result in neurological or physical malfunctioning, while also inhibiting proper circulation of oxygen and spinal fluids around the brain.

Cranial manipulation by a professional therapist involves the application of the correct amount of pressure to the plates, thus allowing for proper motion along the sutures. This increases the flow of oxygen and spinal fluid, and allows for improved neurological functioning.

Cranial-Sacral Therapy

Similar to cranial manipulation, cranial-sacral therapy uses a lighter touch to stimulate the body's natural ability to heal. By balancing the flow of fluid from the cranium to the sacrum at the base of the spine, this gentle adjustment to the nervous system releases healthy energy to the entire body, including the internal organs.

Lymphatic Drainage

Lymph nodes act as the filter system for the body's cells. The lymphatic system cleanses inorganic toxins, cell wastes, excess water, microorganisms, and other components. A light, relaxing massage serves to drain the lymphatic system of impurities, allowing them to leave the body.

Massage

One of the oldest forms of healing, massage brings deep relaxation and comfort to the body and mind. Our staff members are experts in shiatsu, reflexology, and Swedish massage.

Spinal Manipulation and Structural Alignment

Manual manipulation of the vertebrae and musculature helps create proper alignment of the spine.

Clay Therapies

Clay Packs

Luvos clay, imported from Germany, is used for the deep cleansing of the liver and other affected areas. The drying action of the wet clay draws toxins out of the organs and brings them to the skin's surface where they can be absorbed into the clay.

Fango Treatment

Prepared from medicinal clay imported from Germany, fango high-intensity heat packs are applied in order to relax and detoxify the body. Fango applications cover large sections of the body, such as the back, chest, shoulders, or legs.

Ginger Packs

To increase circulation to the legs and lower extremities, packs of ginger may be applied to stimulate vitality and reduce congestion. If applied over the navel and kept warm, it soothes the stomach; if done in conjunction with acupuncture, it can help rebuild the adrenal glands. This treatment is prescribed for all blood types.

Hot Packs

Applied in cases of muscular spasm, hot packs work to establish proper circulation.

Oxygen Therapies

Hyperbaric Oxygen Machine

This therapeutic equipment provides a rich, rejuvenating, and reviving supply of oxygen to deprived cells. The aim is to speed healing, while increasing overall energy and circulation. Additional benefits include fighting premature aging, destroying abnormal cells, and providing oxygen to cells that have been starved due to multiple sclerosis and other neurological disorders.

Infrared Sauna with Oxygen

Typical saunas heat the body from the outside, concentrating on the skin. This specialized sauna applies heat to the internal tissues by emitting far-infrared energy that penetrates the skin and directly heats subcutaneous fat layers. This type of sauna has been proven very effective in helping the body eliminate heavy metals and other toxins that lie beneath the skin.

Multistep Therapy

Our staff carefully monitors your condition as you breathe in pure oxygen and gently pedal a specially designed stationary bicycle. This double stimulation brings life-giving oxygen to the brain and circulatory system, promoting proper circulation throughout the body.

Specialized Therapies

Color, Music, and Negative-Ion Therapy

The institute's therapeutic use of color, music, and negative ions produces a deeply calming sensation, providing a highly effective and thoroughly enjoyable antidote to stress.

Cupping

This ancient therapy originally involved glass cups with candles, used as suction devices, to increase blood flow to a particular area, such as the chest cavity or the back. Today, we use machines to produce the same effect.

Diapulse

Designed to create pulsed non-thermal electromagnetic energy, this unique machine is a valuable tool for increasing blood supply to damaged or diseased areas, thereby stimulating repair.

Diathermy

This heat-producing apparatus is used to increase circulation, decrease inflammation, and stimulate healing in injured tissue.

Firard Therapy

The Firard machine offers yet another option when deep, penetrating heat is desired. It generates far-infrared light waves that aren't stopped at the body's surface as are conventional infrared waves. This machine is often used to stimulate acupuncture needles in the treatment of lower-back pain or to increase "yang" energy in the body.

G-5 Vibration Treatments

This treatment is designed to produce intense vibrations that relax tense and strained muscles, and improve circulation.

Intravenous (IV) Infusion

Administered by a naturopathic doctor, our IV infusion bathes internal cells and tissues with substances that increase overall energy, improve the strength of the immune system, and perform actions targeted to various conditions. This is one of the institute's most powerful tools in speeding the healing process. Our IVs are unique in that they contain mixtures of vitamins specifically blended for the individual blood type of the patient.

Iontophoresis Therapy

This painless, nonintrusive treatment uses a galvanic current on the skin to encourage the penetration of an assortment of topical applications, thereby helping to relieve pain.

Laser Therapy

This sophisticated laser therapy is used to improve circulation in areas of congestion or inflammation of bone or tissue.

Light Therapy

NASA research has shown that light therapy decreases wound healing time. It is believed to increase the overall energy available to the cells, which stimulates fibroblasts to produce collagen, the protein that makes connective tissue. Light therapy is used to treat injuries, reduce pain and inflammation, and reinforce the energy generated during acupuncture.

Magnetic-Field Therapy

When your body is placed in the center of a magnetic field, hydrogen and oxygen molecules are caused to join in the cell. Metabolism is increased, stimulating the cell to eliminate carbon dioxide and replace it with oxygen. This helps rid the body of cells that have been damaged by degenerative diseases.

Myosynchrone

Gentle energy pulses are used to increase circulation and relax the musculature. This treatment is often used in conjunction with hydrotherapy.

TensCam

All living creatures on Earth—and the Earth itself—typically resonate at a frequency of 7.86 Hz. Where there is inflammation, congestion, or diseased tissue, natural energy is drained and the frequency drops. The TensCam generates electromagnetic "tens" waves that pass through a specially attuned crystal transducer to become scalar waves. This energy is directed into the body toward areas of decreased resonance, restoring the area to its natural frequency. This change facilitates the body's innate healing powers.

Ultrasound Therapy

The ultrasound device emits sound waves beyond the range of human hearing. These waves readily penetrate the body, stimulating and massaging the cells and tissues below the skin in such a way as to generate heat and increase circulation. A gel is applied to the area prior to treatment to facilitate penetration. The gel has been impregnated with herbal substances, and the waves help these ingredients pass through the skin. They can then work their healing actions directly on damaged tissues and help break down calcium deposits in the body.

ACKNOWLEDGMENTS

Thank you to my daughter, Dr. Michele D'Adamo, for all of her hard work and support in writing this book. I would also like to thank my patients who have contributed to my research and have submitted many of the recipes that appear in this book.

Allan Richards thanks Alice N. Monro, his energetic and multi-tasking researcher/editorial assistant for her perspicacity and hard work.

ABOUT THE AUTHOR

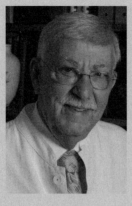 **Dr. James L. D'Adamo, N.D. D.N.B.**, is the originator of the world-famous Blood-Type Diet and director of the D'Adamo Institute for the Advancement of Natural Therapies. Trained in the United States, Germany, and Switzerland, Dr. D'Adamo revolutionized natural medicine more than 50 years ago with his discovery of the correlation between people's blood type and their dietary and exercise requirements. His landmark books, *One Man's Food... is someone else's poison* (1980) and *The D'Adamo Diet* (1989), rejected standardized approaches of treatment and passionately called for diagnosis and care based on the individual.

Dr. D'Adamo began his practice in New York and has also worked in London, Montreal, Antwerp, and Chihuahua, Mexico, treating over 50,000 patients, including many celebrities. He currently works at offices in Portsmouth, New Hampshire; and Toronto, Canada, where he and his team of naturopathic specialists provide the most comprehensive natural health care in North America.

Allan Richards collaborated with Dr. D'Adamo on his groundbreaking book *One Man's Food . . . is someone else's poison*. He was a judge for the Scripps Howard 2009 National Journalism Awards and was awarded a 2009 Kaiser Mini-Fellowship for Global Health Reporting on HIV/AIDS in South Africa. Richards is an associate professor and the interim associate dean of Florida International University's School of Journalism and Mass Communication in Miami.

www.dadamoinstitute.com

D'Adamo Institute	D'Adamo Institute
44 Bridge Street	186 St. George Street
Portsmouth, NH	Toronto, Ontario,
03801-3902	Canada M5R 2N3
(603) 430-7600	(416) 968-0496

We hope you enjoyed this Hay House book.
If you would like to receive a free catalogue featuring additional
Hay House books and products, or if you would like information
about the Hay Foundation, please contact:

Hay House UK Ltd
292B Kensal Road • London W10 5BE
Tel: (44) 20 8962 1230; Fax: (44) 20 8962 1239
www.hayhouse.co.uk

***

Published and distributed in the United States of America by:
Hay House, Inc. • PO Box 5100 • Carlsbad, CA 92018-5100
Tel: (1) 760 431 7695 or (1) 800 654 5126;
Fax: (1) 760 431 6948 or (1) 800 650 5115
www.hayhouse.com

***

Published and distributed in Australia by:
Hay House Australia Ltd • 18/36 Ralph Street • Alexandria, NSW 2015
Tel: (61) 2 9669 4299, Fax: (61) 2 9669 4144
www.hayhouse.com.au

***

Published and distributed in the Republic of South Africa by:
Hay House SA (Pty) Ltd • PO Box 990 • Witkoppen 2068
Tel/Fax: (27) 11 467 8904
www.hayhouse.co.za

***

Published and distributed in India by:
Hay House Publishers India • Muskaan Complex • Plot No.3
B-2• Vasant Kunj • New Delhi - 110 070
Tel: (91) 11 41761620; Fax: (91) 11 41761630
www.hayhouse.co.in

***

Distributed in Canada by:
Raincoast • 9050 Shaughnessy St • Vancouver, BC V6P 6E5
Tel: (1) 604 323 7100
Fax: (1) 604 323 2600

***

Sign up via the Hay House UK website to receive the Hay House
online newsletter and stay informed about what's going on with your
favourite authors. You'll receive bimonthly announcements
about discounts and offers, special events, product highlights,
free excerpts, giveaways, and more!
www.hayhouse.co.uk

Mind Your Body,
Mend Your Spirit

Hay House is the ultimate resource for inspirational and health-conscious books, audio programs, movies, events, e-newsletters, member communities, and much more.

Visit **www.hayhouse.com**® today and nourish your soul.

UPLIFTING EVENTS
Join your favorite authors at live events in a city near you or log on to **www.hayhouse.com** to visit with Hay House authors online during live, interactive Web events.

INSPIRATIONAL RADIO
Daily inspiration while you're at work or at home. Enjoy radio programs featuring your favorite authors, streaming live on the Internet 24/7 at **HayHouseRadio.com**®. Tune in and tune up your spirit!

VIP STATUS
Join the Hay House VIP membership program today and enjoy exclusive discounts on books, CDs, calendars, card decks, and more. You'll also receive 10% off all event reservations (excluding cruises). Visit **www.hayhouse.com/wisdom** to join the Hay House Wisdom Community™.

Visit **www.hayhouse.com** and enter priority code 2723 during checkout for special savings!
(One coupon per customer.)

JOIN THE HAY HOUSE FAMILY

As the leading self-help, mind, body and spirit publisher in the UK, we'd like to welcome you to our family so that you can enjoy all the benefits our website has to offer.

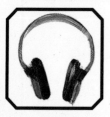 **EXTRACTS** from a selection of your favourite author titles

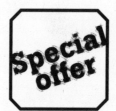 **COMPETITIONS, PRIZES & SPECIAL OFFERS** Win extracts, money off, downloads and so much more

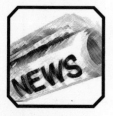 **LISTEN** to a range of radio interviews and our latest audio publications

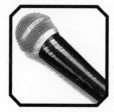 **CELEBRATE YOUR BIRTHDAY** An inspiring gift will be sent your way

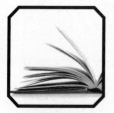 **LATEST NEWS** Keep up with the latest news from and about our authors

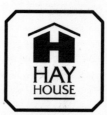 **ATTEND OUR AUTHOR EVENTS** Be the first to hear about our author events

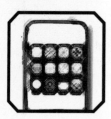 **iPHONE APPS** Download your favourite app for your iPhone

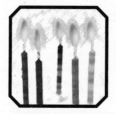 **HAY HOUSE INFORMATION** Ask us anything, all enquiries answered

join us online at **www.hayhouse.co.uk**

 292B Kensal Road, London W10 5BE
T: 020 8962 1230 E: info@hayhouse.co.uk